Angels of Mercy

An Eyewitness Account of Civil War
and Yellow Fever

by a Sister of Mercy

Regards,
Sister M. Paulinus

A primary source by
Sister Ignatius Sumner, R.S.M.

Author/Editor
Sister Mary Paulinus Oakes, R.S.M.

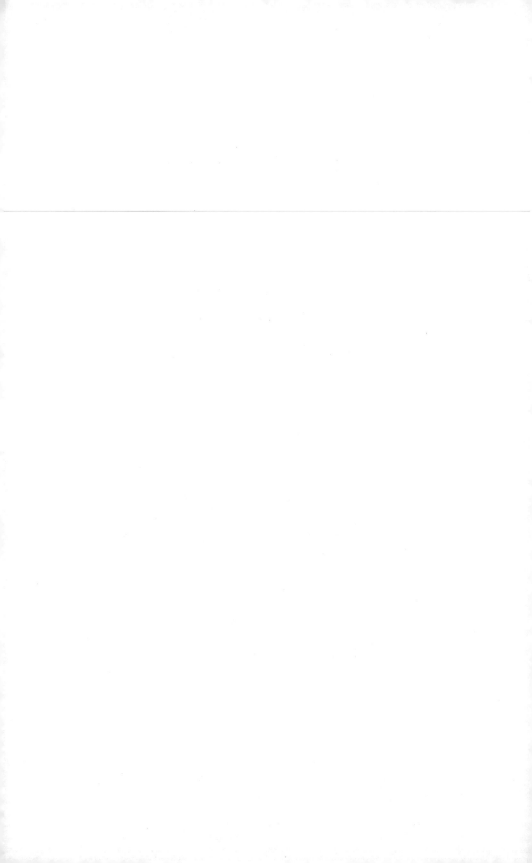

Printed and bound in the United States of America

3 4 5   12 11 10 09 08 07 06 05 04 03 02 01 99 98 97

ISBN 1-885938-12-8

Library of Congress Catalog Card Number: 98-070216

Published in 1998
Second Printing 2000
Third Printing 2012

Cathedral Foundation Press
P.O. Box 777
Baltimore, Maryland 21203

Publisher: Christopher Gunty
Book and cover design: Karen Pellegrini
Production assistant: Karen Pellegrini
Printing: Catholic Printing Solutions, Baltimore, MD

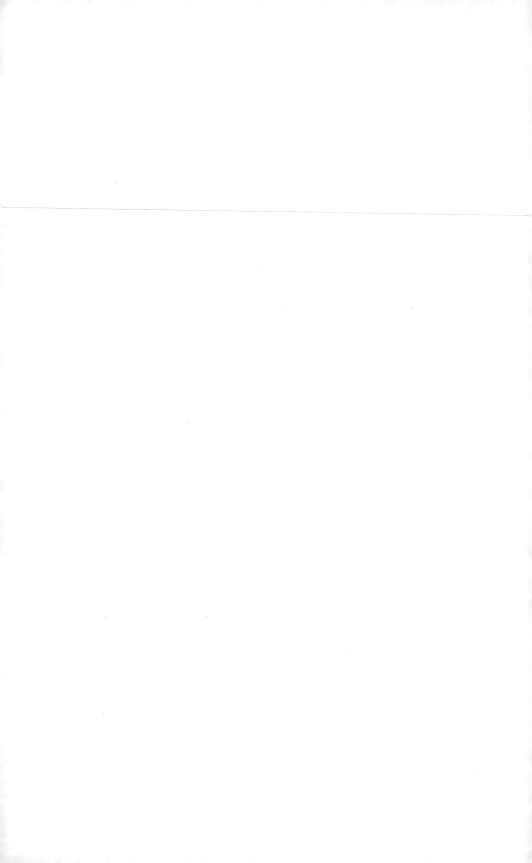

Table of Contents

DEDICATION

To the more than 300 Sisters of Mercy who have ministered in Mississippi since 1860 and to the bishops who have co-ministered with them.

To the present Sisters of Mercy and Associates serving in the state.

May God continue to bless Mercy efforts in education, health care, and in meeting the emerging needs of those most dispossessed and marginalized in our society. May all Mercies follow the early examples of Sister DeSales Browne and Bishop Henry Elder in new and flexible ways of serving those most in need.

To those who sensed the importance of what was happening and who preserved precious accounts of the past we owe our gratitude. The recordings of Sister Ignatius Sumner, Bishop William Henry Elder, Bishop Richard Gerow and Sister Angela Fedou have helped establish deep roots and pride in our past as church members, Sisters of Mercy, and Mississippians in the noblest sense.

ACKNOWLEDGEMENTS

Sister Callista Reddoch, deceased, was most anxious to see this work published. Without her encouragement and that of Sister Mary Emmanuel Harper, present archivist, of the Sisters of Mercy Vicksburg, publication would never have been possible. Over this ten year period of editing Sister Emmanuel has been untiring in her efforts at aiding with research. Sister Callista had the expanded diary typed by Catherine Williamson and Anna Claire Gamble. They worked tirelessly on this important document and expansion of this journal. Typists who typed from the original manuscript deserve thanks: Sister Joan Maureen Landry and Glenda LaGarde; many others typed at different stages: Susan Casper, Marye Lou Lee, Freida McElleheny, Rhonda Dunigan, Russell Dyer, and finally Louise Cox. Thanks to numerous readers and critics: Sister Mary Anne O'Brien, Sister Carolyn Zionce, Sister Timothy Matthews, Sister Dorothy Loeb, Carol Weimar, Dolores Salmon, Dorothy Taylor. Sister Elise Todd and Sister Mary Matthew McCloskey both had done extensive research in 1960; their research and their advice and support were most helpful. Advice was solicited from Dr. John Marsalek, Mississippi State University; Dr. Frank Allen Dennis, Delta State; Morris Raphael, author New Iberia; Christopher Kauffman, author, Catholic University; Brother Thomas Spalding CFX, Spalding College, author and historian, expert on "Frontier Catholicism"!

Ken Penhale of Shelby Springs, Alabama became a friend when he was one of the originators of the research on the Shelby Springs hospital and cemetery. He has been a constant supporter. Yearly his historical society has commemorated the Sisters' contribution by monuments and memorials. His society refurbished the cemetery and made it a tourist attraction. Each year the Sisters have been invited to participate in the annual Confederate Memorial Day event; this has been an encouragement to publish the journal. Their memorial to Father Leray prompted me to do more research and include a biography of him in the Addendum to the journal. Ken also provided photographs.

Gordon Cotton has been another encourager and mentor. His continuing dialogue over a number of years has made me appreciative of the vast history of St. Francis convent and school and the Sisters contribution to the history of Vicksburg. Gordon shared documents of the

Court Martial of the Minerva Cook murderers and his own book *THE MURDER OF MINERVA HYNES COOK*. He has been an invaluable source on every aspect of local history.

Charles Riles has been a friend of the Sisters and has buried many at no cost as owner of Fisher-Riles Funeral Home. He has done extensive research on each Sister and made a scrapbook of obituaries. This has been a priceless resource.

Sister Ethelbert Demuth, deceased, did her master's thesis on the history of the Sisters of Mercy and St. Francis School from 1860-1960. She interviewed a number of the senior Sisters and recorded important information in this thesis. Several of the Sisters remembered Sister De-Sales and related some interesting tales. Sister Ethelbert was originally from Omaha but fell in love with St. Francis School and Convent and all its history. She was a dear friend and companion; her enthusiasm for our history and her research were contagious.

Brother Thomas Spalding, CFX, proofread the entire manuscript and biographies and made corrections and suggestions. The input of a historian of his stature was indeed appreciated. His cousin Joanne Boone Bellan proofed a later version, as did Eileen Payne. A final reading with accurate historical corrections and additions was done by Edwin C. Bearrs, noted historian and author.

Footnotes have been included on each page of the journal for clarity's sake and easier reading. Because eleven pages of the journal were missing, and Sister Ignatius dictated those years later in the expanded journal, the original does not follow chronological order. I have tried to be as true as possible to the primary source, thus footnotes on the pages. The biographies are addendum but necessary I believe to enflesh the whole scene and complete the history of the time and place. Endnotes are at the end of the book for the biographies.

Editor's Introduction

As a child growing up in Vicksburg, Mississippi, in the 1930's, and attending St. Francis School, I became imbued with the Civil War history of the place. Our kindergarten building had been a hospital for the wounded. One of the early Sister principals, a Vicksburger, Sister Margaret Mary Kearney, had been born in a cave during the shelling of the city. Also born in a cave was the Mississippi historian Sister Bernard Maguire. U. S. Grant's forces occupied my school and would not relinquish the property when the Sisters made efforts to reclaim it.

My mind could not fathom anyone not cooperating with, much less defying, the Sisters whom I so greatly admired and loved. The first young woman to be received as a Sister of Mercy in Vicksburg during the war, Sister Xavier Poursine, had taught my mother as a small child. I remember the last Confederate Veteran who died in Vicksburg, Jim Bitterman, who had been a young drummer boy and recounted wonderful stories to me as a child.

There was an aura about the buildings themselves, the school and convent, a sacred history so to speak. Over 200 graduates dedicated their lives as Sisters of Mercy in the chapel, taking their vows of service to the poor, sick, and uneducated. Much of the furniture there had withstood the siege and had been donated by families, some by Jefferson Davis' own family. There were cannon shells in the school display cases. In the hall there was a beautiful Sacred Heart statue given in gratitude to the Sisters for having nursed the Yellow Fever victims in Edwards, Mississippi in 1898, since the Sisters would not accept a monetary gift.

A large part of my culture, my heritage and my religious experience was caught up in the history of the place. As I remember most of it was oral history. I was one of the 200 local Mississippians who throughout the years joined the Sisters of Mercy and served in several of the twenty Mississippi Mercy institutions numbered among countless others in the United States and throughout the English speaking world.

I was privileged to serve in the illustrious line of principals of my alma mater. The author of the journal presented here was the first principal; the second, Sister Angela Fedou, served forty-three years and died in the principal's office. This was indicative of the kind of Mercy dedication.

The oral tradition continued to be handed down. Alumni had fierce loyalties; children sang hymns composed by the Sisters; they wrote essays on local history; they did interviews, the traditions were preserved. Wonderful stories were told of the deeds of the deceased Sisters. Scholars who came to the archives to write history included an author, Barbara Roberts, a group of historians from Shelby Springs, Alabama, where the Sisters had nursed the last three years of the war, and an anthropologist, Ralph Bishop, from Chicago on a Humanities grant. Our own alumna, Glenda LaGarde, a Mercy historian in her own right and a fourth generation alumna and supporter of the school, secured another Humanities grant to study the life and history of the school and its influence on the community. Glenda delved into the archives for information; they were a treasure of history.

I became more interested and researched the archives following her example. Here I discovered the annals of the Sisters of Mercy from various areas of our country and Ireland and England. I read of the Sisters' participation in the Crimean War, with both English and Irish Sisters helping Florence Nightingale, and the American Sisters, vast participation in all arenas of the Civil War. I read George Barton's *Angels of the Battlefield* (1898), where he attempted to give some history of the activities of the Catholic Sisterhoods during this war. His thesis was to fill in the historical gap in the published literature of the war which had totally neglected or barely mentioned the self-sacrificing labors of the Sisters.

In researching historical documents and primary sources from archives in Vicksburg and information from archives of the Sisters of Mercy throughout the county, I was astonished to learn of the quantity and quality of the Sisters' services during the Civil War, subsequent wars, and the Yellow Fever and influenza epidemics. The Sisters of Mercy nursed the wounded in the rotunda of the nation's capitol even as work progressed on the Great Dome. Sister Ignatius' journal tells of the Sisters' similar nursing exploits here in Mississippi's capitol building. My favorite portrait is the one President Abraham Lincoln commissioned. Grant described the scene to Lincoln of the Sister in Vicksburg administering to a dying soldier and Lincoln pointing to some of the Sisters of the Baltimore and New York Communities doing duty in Washington. Lincoln then sent for the White House artist, Florence Meyer to depict the scene on canvas. Both Jefferson Davis and Abraham Lincoln paid tribute to the Sisters. Wrote Davis: "I can never forget your kindness to the sick and wounded during our darkest days. And I know not how to testify my gratitude and respect for every member of your noble order."

Lincoln said much the same: "Of all the forms of charity and benevolence seen in the crowded wards of the hospitals, those of the Catholic sisters were among the most efficient.... As they went from cot to cot distributing the medicines prescribed, or administering the cooling, strengthening draughts as directed, they were veritable angels of mercy."

Lincoln possibly well remembered the incident in Washington in the Douglas Hospital where a Sister of Mercy, experiencing total exasperation and righteous anger with lack of food for the wounded, went over the heads of the bureaucrats in the War Department directly to Lincoln, and he gave a written presidential order that Sisters of Mercy be given exactly what they requested for the sick and wounded and that it be charged to the War Department.

During the time of my intense research in 1991, seventeen regional Mercy congregations united to form one congregation, the Institute of the Sisters of Mercy of the Americas. The Institute includes 6,700 Sisters of Mercy and 1,400 Mercy Associates. There is a worldwide membership of more than 15,000 Sisters. This union strengthened the order to continue to carry out the mission of the foundress, Catherine McAuley, of Dublin, Ireland, in 1831: quality service to the poor, sick, and uneducated, especially women and children.

A remarkable woman of compassion and prayer, Catherine McAuley was a socialite, a lady of fashion who chose to live among the poor, a woman of wealth who gave away her money and practiced the discipline of sanctity. She lived the biblical quote, "Whatsoever you do to the least of my people that you do unto me," and she left this as her legacy to the largest community of religious women in the English-speaking world. Born to a wealthy family, she tasted bitter poverty when her father died. As an adult, she regained wealthy adoptive parents, fervent Quakers, with whom she learned to love and share the Scriptures. She was an ecumenical woman before her time. From early childhood, she was drawn to helping the poor in Ireland and used her inherited fortune to practice the works of mercy.

Others joined her, and the Catholic Church called her to begin a religious order. She insisted on a fourth vow to add to poverty, celibacy, and obedience, the traditional vows: a commitment to the works of mercy, service to the poor, sick and uneducated and those wounded by contemporary society. The Mercy Rule was one of the first ever approved by the Catholic Church to give the Sisters the freedom to be wherever the poor, the sick, and the uneducated needed help. Catherine McAuley was an active nun before active nuns. The Irish lovingly referred to the Sisters as the "Moving Nuns," and move they did all over the English-speaking world. The growth of the order was phenomenal even before the order had Church approval. In 1828 Catherine brought home the first abandoned sick child whose parents had died of influenza. Fifteen years later in 1843 seven Sisters of Mercy came to Pittsburgh for the first American Foundation. Just 23 years later, in 1860, a group of six "Moving Nuns" came to Vicksburg from Baltimore. The River City was a den of vice; chaos prevailed; a young doctor had been killed by gamblers; prostitution was rampant. Vicksburg was a microcosm of Mississippi, a very coarse society. Vicksburgers wanted a Christian education and some cultural influences for their children.

One of the six Sisters who came to Mississippi was an American version of Catherine McAuley herself, Sister Ignatius Sumner. This wealthy Baltimore socialite was an accomplished musician with the best teaching credentials and education that the East had to offer. In editing this work I have come to venerate Sister Ignatius as I have read and reread her writings, and as I have researched the various personages she mentions. I have read and reread Bishop Elder's journal, a very matter-of-fact piece of writing, which verifies and expands many incidents recorded by Sister.

I have researched Sister's family, and I was touched by her humility especially by her personal scrapbook. The little that was there whetted my curiosity for what was not there: letters between her and her mother, between the Sisters in Baltimore, her brothers, her sisters and her uncle, the powerful, Massachusetts Senator Charles Sumner. The journal is so typical of convent life — someone borrows several pages and fails to replace them and this gap is left. In her old age she recounts from memory the missing events to a young Sister, thus a gap in chronology.

What I have pieced together of her biography, her mother's and her Jesuit brothers, and what she shows of herself in the journal is the portrait of a woman of the nineteenth century. Her family was steeped in American history. She was truly a valiant woman. We are indebted to Sister Ignatius for her writings which provide us with a deeper view into our Mercy history. The city of Vicksburg purchased the convent and school buildings and have named the city block the Southern Cultural Heritage Center. Plans are to rehabilitate the facility and operate it as an artistic, cultural and programming center in Vicksburg in co-operation with the Center for the Study of Southern Culture at the University of Mississippi.

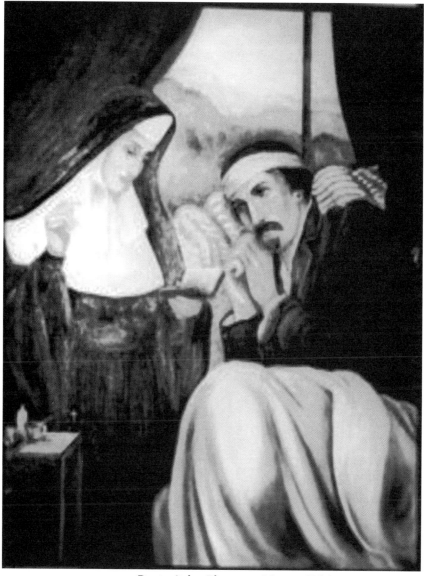

Portrait by Florence Meyer, White House Artist
"The Catholic Sisters were the most efficient...veritable Angels of Mercy."
–President Abraham Lincoln

Sister Ignatius Sumner
c. 1825-1895

Witnessing the shelling of Vicksburg, nursing wounded in the newly established school, following major Civil War battles, traveling a three-state area by railroad box cars with wounded, praying with dying soldiers are all vividly described in the journal of Sister Ignatius Sumner. She gives accounts of the significant daily happenings from 1860, when she and her five companions arrived in Vicksburg, until her death from malaria fever in 1895. This pioneer Mercy nun records events of the yellow fever saga where one half of the population is decimated including deaths of six of her dearest Sister companions, and parish priests, and the Bishop was mistakenly reported dead. She, the excellent teacher, was loaned to the group to start an outstanding educational institution; she reports with frankness, candor, humility, humor. This teacher turned wartime reporter and nurse mentions very little of herself. What is between the lines speaks volumes. Years afterwards, she tries patiently to re-construct parts of the journal from memory after pages have been carelessly lost. She sensed "that the record, the only one, may be interesting to our Sisters at some future time if preserved."

After 70 years of living life "in war and rumor of war" pestilence, pain sorrow and the cross, writing and teaching, Sister Ignatius ironically dies from malaria fever. Her life was a constant paradox; her ministry a greater paradox. Sister Austin Carroll, Mercy historian and contemporary, states that "perhaps no other community ever had so many obstacles in its incipient stages."[1]

This teacher turned nurse downed by a fever! What a paradox to live through the bloody Civil War to spend nights acting as a human tourniquet – this sensitive lady of the 19th century a mix of gentleness and toughness; detachment, survival; a giver of compassion, a recipient of callous prejudice. This genteel cultured lady, gifted musician, writer, steeped in literature, a woman with the best education America could provide in the 19th century in the Arts; this talented teacher spends her energies on the battlefields of the Civil War doing rudimentary nursing. Fingers cultivated for the piano used to cover the bleeding artery of a teenage soldier. This woman of lofty education, genteel and refined, spends her days visiting the poor – crowded homes of immigrants on the levee, cooking and delivering soup to their sick, defending the right of the Irish shanty-boat youngsters to attend school with their lace-curtain countrymen. This well-read lady spends countless hours visiting and consoling prisoners of the city jail. The social outcasts of her time were instructed by word and example in the rudiments of Christian living. With an unusual zest for life and the beauties of music, art and literature, she spends her peak years consoling many a soldier on his deathbed, sharing her rations, preparing bodies for burial.

The Maryland annals tell us that "the hardships that this group of Sisters endured cannot be estimated this side of eternity." Though very hungry herself Sister Ignatius would say, "Let's pray like there is something to eat."[2]

The funeral home records in Vicksburg show that as treasurer of the frugal community she spent money on many shrouds for men, women and children to be buried with some shred of dignity. Besides bathing the brows of those dying with fever, praying and consoling the dying and their survivors, she assumed the responsibility of providing for twenty orphans whose every family member had died in the pestilence of 1878.

What were the roots of this valiant nineteenth century Christian woman? Sister Ignatius was born Frances Sumner, to a Unitarian family whose religious origins dated back to sturdy Puritan stock from Massachusetts, Cotton Mather being an early ancestor as well as Increase Sumner, the 1797 governor of Massachusetts.[3] Her great uncle, Henry Payson, a devout Unitarian, built the church in Baltimore where a memorial bust of him still stands in the church on Franklin Street and Charles Street. Jared Sparks and William Ellery Channing's busts are also prominent in this historical edifice. Henry Payson came to Baltimore during the Revolutionary War. He was influential in raising money and fortifying Baltimore. He and his associates were responsible for repulsing the British at Fort McHenry in 1814 and at the Battle of North Point thus saving the city of Baltimore. These British troops had defeated Napoleon and were ready for an American takeover. They had marched on Washington, soundly defeating the Americans there while President James Madison watched the invasion of the mansion and the destruction of other public buildings. This heroic strategic Battle of North Point drove the British from the east coast and brought the War of 1812 to a conclusion. He later helped to found the Baltimore Stock Exchange. A street is named in memory of this prominent citizen and patriot. Her father, Henry Sumner, was from Roxbury, Massachusetts. He served in the War of 1812 and in the Battle of North Point in 1814.

Her mother was Frances Steele, daughter of John Steele, leading merchant of Baltimore in 1800. Frances Steele was the adopted daughter of Henry Payson, her uncle. Charles Sumner, the leading abolitionist of the era, was Sister Ignatius' uncle, her father's eldest brother.[4] Another uncle, Horace Sumner, participated in the Brook Farm experiment of the Transcendentalists and was drowned in a ship accident off New Jersey near Fire Island while returning from Italy with Margaret Fuller, the renowned American author.[5] Frances' husband, Henry Sumner, died and left Frances a widow at age 38. She had borne nine children, five of whom survived to adulthood. She turned to religion for comfort. Through reading, studying and finally, through the faith and example of her Catholic servants, she became a Catholic. For this, she was alienated from her friends, derided by relatives, and disinherited by her uncle, although he remembered her children in his will. One by one her children followed her example and became Catholics. Her two sons, John and William Sumner became Jesuit priests in the Maryland Province.[6]

How unfortunate that no letters have been preserved. From Jesuit obituaries and biographies it is noted that both brothers were popular teachers and esteemed members of the Society. Their students "held them in great affection and admiration."[7]

John, the eldest sibling, was born in 1819 in Baltimore. When the mother and family converted to the Catholic faith, John was in his teens and unconvinced of Catholicism. He was indignant at his mother's having the children baptized, especially William and Helen since he thought they should be allowed to choose for themselves when older. He remained close to his Unitarian pastor, Jared Sparks, the noted historian. Sparks' bust is also in the Unitarian Church. At his ordination William Ellery Channing gave a two-hour address defining American Unitarianism. Later Sparks became president of Harvard. They were lifelong friends even after he chose for himself to become Catholic and join the Jesuits. Archbishop Martin Spalding asked him to gather the literary men of the day so he could meet them. John brought Henry Wadsworth Longfellow and his uncle, Charles Sumner, to dine at Sparks' dinner table where the Archbishop joined them. As a young man, he served as librarian at the Mercantile Library in Baltimore, one of the best libraries in the United States. He contributed articles to the *Southern Literary Messenger*, possibly the leading magazine in America. He entered the Jesuits in 1856 at the age of thirty-seven, one year after his sister entered the Sisters of Mercy. He co-edited the *Messenger of the Sacred Heart* and started the *Georgetown College Journal*. A popular teacher, John served at St. Joseph College, Philadelphia, Holy Cross and Georgetown. His obituary in the Journal was written with great grief by one of his students who affectionately describes his "venerable tobacco-box which he shared bountifully with students." He died suddenly in 1880, preceding his mother in death by two years. William administered the last rites. John is buried in the old Georgetown cemetery.[8]

William, second boy, and fourth sibling, was born in 1834; he was a civil engineer and a French scholar. As a young man he served as an official in the Baltimore Post Office and was 25 when he entered the Jesuits in 1859, three years after his brother. Undoubtedly, Sister Ignatius' entrance to the Sisters of Mercy had profound influence on both brothers.

William was one of the founders of the Maryland Historical Society. He did a family genealogy and was probably instrumental in re-establishing ties with Charles Sumner. He spent fourteen years at Georgetown as French teacher. He waited sixteen years before ordination because of his humility and his awe of the priesthood. Interestingly, the year 1867-68, William spent in Spring Hill College, Mobile, for health reasons. Surely he was able to visit Sister Ignatius at this time. He taught at Gonzaga College and Boston College for short stints. Back at Georgetown he was superior of junior scholastics and served his last 13 years at St. Ignatius Church while also teaching. Here he was a most popular confessor. He died in 1905 and was buried at Woodstock.[9]

Surely these two brothers were an integral part of Sister Ignatius' life. However, there are only a few incidents where any contact is recorded. They were generous contributors to the Sisters in Vicksburg, giving an oil painting of the crucifixion, and the altar in the convent chapel. It is believed they used their influence to get the convent back from the United States after the war. John directed one very talented young lady, Frances Kelly from Baltimore to enter the order in Vicksburg with Sister Ignatius as her mentor. She became Sister Regis and was a fine artist. Probably both brothers directed other promising young ladies to the Vicksburg foundation since the records show many young women from Baltimore entering at that period. During the Yellow Fever epidemic in 1878, the school closed for six months and the journal indicates that the Sisters would have been unable to subsist without donations from the Sisters' relatives.[10]

Sister Ignatius had two sisters, Valerie and Helen. Valerie, the oldest daughter and second sibling, married a man named Williams and was widowed at the time of her mother's death in 1882. Helen was the youngest, a year younger than William.[11] She figured prominently in her sister's life and in U. S. history. Helen came to Vicksburg and served as fund raiser for the school after the war. She put on numerous plays and city-wide pageants to entertain the people of Vicksburg and raised money for the school buildings which had been stripped and vandalized, thus freeing the Sisters to teach and practice the works of Mercy. The expanded journal tells that in 1867 she had a series of tableaus and a fair which raised $4,500, a remarkable sum because of floods and crop failure. The Sisters bought a piece of ground adjacent to the original building to erect the convent and additional rooms for the school.

Helen's obituary in 1887 is informative:

She nursed the wounded on the field

Mrs. Helen Sumner Bradford, aged fifty-two, wife of Jef-
ferson Davis Bradford, died on Sunday at midnight. Her
mother-in-law was Amanda J. Davis Bradford, a sister of
Jefferson Davis. Mrs. Helen Bradford was the daughter of
the late Henry P. Sumner and grandniece of Henry Payson.
She was an ardent Southerner and nursed the wounded on
the Gettysburg battlefield. Funeral from the Cathedral at
9:30 Tuesday morning. [12]

In her scrapbook, Sister Ignatius had a tiny wedding card announcing:

St. Peter's Church Half-Past 8 o'clock, p.m. Tuesday, July
21, 1868
Jeff D. Bradford   Helen P. Sumner [13]

Helen and Jeff lived in Yonkers, New York. At the request of Sister Ignatius, after the war, the couple took at least one young Southern girl whose family had been impoverished by the War and helped educate her in the same manner as their family had been educated. The girl was Clara Juliene of Jackson, Mississippi, who later entered the Sisters of Mercy and became Sister Margaret Mary, an accomplished musician and teacher. [14] Another entry in Sister Ignatius' scrapbook must have been the marriage of Helen and Jeff's son. Only this:

*Virginia Patterson to Colonel J. D. Bradford of
Indian Territory marriage in St. Matthew's
by Father Sumner.*[15]

Another famous relative was Charles Sumner of Massachusetts fame. He was an ardent abolitionist of the time and an avid advocate of public education and prison reform. Charles Sumner could be abrasive in defense of his causes and suffered greatly from being beaten with a cane in the Senate by an opponent, Preston Brooks of South Carolina. He was nephew of Senator Andrew Butler, advocate of the Kansas-Nebraska Act. Charles Sumner and Henry, Sister's father had a family argument before Henry's marriage. Thus began their open enmity; they never spoke to each other again.[16] Sister never mentioned Charles Sumner in her journal, but she had a picture of him and Henry Wadsworth Longfellow in her scrapbook. Her brother re-established family and social ties much later in Baltimore.[17] Sister Ignatius certainly shared Charles' tenacity and ability to see injustice but was blessed with a good sense of humor and her mother's "genial manner" and "unfailing charity."[18] Charles Sumner and Henry Wadsworth Longfellow were close friends. One has to wonder if Charles knew his niece was nursing wounded Confederate soldiers when he penned his congratulations to General William T. Sherman for his victories in Vicksburg and Jackson. When Longfellow penned his tribute to the Sisters of Mercy, did he have his friend's niece in mind when he wrote:

> *Other hope had she none, nor wish in life, but to follow*
> *Meekly, with reverent steps, the sacred feet of her Savior,*
> *And with light in her looks, she entered the chamber of sickness,*
> *Moistening the feverish lip, and the aching brow, and in silence*
> *Closing the sightless eyes of the dead, and concealing their faces,*
> *Where on their pallets they lay, like drifts of snow on the road-*
> *side.*
> *Many a languid head, upraised as the Sister entered,*
> *Turned on its pillow of pain to gaze while she passed, for her*
> *presence Fell on their hearts like a ray of sun on the walls of a*
> *prison.*[19]

In her humility throughout the journal, Sister Ignatius never makes mention of her family. She refers to her blood sister, Helen, as H.S. in the rewritten pages; we later find out it was Helen. Other sources are necessary for family information. No letters were kept, and no picture of her is available. The Maryland Annals describe her as "a distinguished looking woman, tall, graceful, and well-proportioned. She was charmingly dignified in manner and could appear to advantage in any society into which she was introduced." As Sister Ignatius, she was a great favorite with the Sisters in her community because of her sweet amiable disposition.[20]

As Fannie Sumner, she reigned as a belle in the most exclusive Baltimore society. When she entered the Sisters of Mercy in Baltimore, the congregation was young, having been formed from the Pittsburgh group only a few years previously. All had been on the staff of the Washington Infirmary. All were young with the exception of Sister Catherine Wynne, the leader. Later, Sister Camillus, Catherine McAuley's godchild, was sent to help (she was in her mid 30s), and Sister Ligouri was lent to give experienced educational leadership to the young group. Fannie's mother gave her daughter to the Mercy Order with some uncertainties but unfailing faith and humility. In preparing her trousseau to enter the convent, it was required that she bring a wash board. Her mother wrote a note to Sister Catherine Wynne to "Please have patience with my Fannie; she had never had experience with a wash board, but she learns quickly."[21]

At the time she entered, the Sisters were staffing the Washington Infirmary, a teaching hospital with a distinguished faculty of doctors. She was under the spiritual tutelage of Sister Catherine Wynne, the third person to join the Sisters of Mercy in the U.S., and Sister Camillus Byrne. This novitiate consisted of some of the finest women that the community produced. One of Sister Catherine Wynne's gifts was a discernment for fine young women and their training in the Mercy way.

Sister Ignatius, as all of these early members, served her term nursing in the wards of the Washington Infirmary. In 1855 and 1856, she and Sister Vincent Browne and Sister Alphonsus Atkinson were trained together by Sister Camillus Byrne. The latter brought the true spirit of a Sister of Mercy straight from Dublin and from the association with Catherine McAuley who reared and educated her. Sister Camillus was present at the death of Catherine McAuley. She instructed her charges in the visitation of the poor and sick, jail and penitentiary, and the works of mercy dear to the original spirit of the Institute. Sister Catherine Wynne and Sister Camillus were ideal models, a mixture of Mercy prayer and works, ideal to form new aspirants in the Mercy spirit.

Sister Ignatius worked in the Washington Infirmary for a short time, learned the nursing skills of the day, went on to teach at the Academy and later went into fund raising.[22]

Sister Ignatius had been groomed as a teacher at the Academy of Our Lady of Mercy Baltimore. The Academy was opened in 1855 (same year as she entered the community) and attended by daughters of the best families in the city. There was such a large initial enrollment that Sister Ligouri McCaffrey was sent from Pittsburgh to get the school organized and the faculty trained. She had been educated in a first-class academy in Carlow, Ireland and had come to America in 1843 with Mother Xavier Warde and the pioneer American group. The school Sister Ligouri had attended had been opened by Catherine McAuley who had given instructions there to Dr. McCaffrey's three daughters, one of whom was Sister Ligouri. In Pittsburgh, Sister Ligouri was an outstanding school manager and administrator. With this Mercy educator, Sister Ignatius' potential was realized to the maximum. After a very short time, the Archbishop closed the school, so all the Sisters could work in the "poor" parochial school. Within a year, he reopened the academy after realizing that the Sisters of Mercy always followed the example of Catherine McAuley, their foundress, by running academies in order to be able to finance the free schools.

Many of their vocations to the order came from the academies. A hallmark of Mercy from the beginning was networking the rich to the poor. Sister Ignatius was again placed in the academy and given the leadership in soliciting financial aid from friends and relatives for a new building. She was a successful development directress and soon a serviceable building was erected. Along with her talent as a teacher, she was also an adroit fund raiser and accountant.

During these first years, Sister Catherine Wynne was dying of cancer. She was particularly fond of Sister Ignatius. They had shared many an early hardship. Catherine had come to Baltimore, one of the largest cities in the country, with three companions and no money. She had been given an empty shell of a building for a school. She states: "Many a time have I walked up and down the empty rooms, wondering within myself where the necessary furniture was to be procured, or whence the next meal was to come".[23]

God sent her the enthusiastic, energetic, talented Fanny Sumner, who had a penchant for raising funds, endearing herself to her fellow sisters, and who charmed Archbishop Kenrick into reopening the Academy.

Now the Archbishop made a request for a group to go to the Vicksburg, Mississippi, territory. With so few Sisters how could this take place? What a heroic response to say, "yes," to the request. What a poignant thought to separate. Catherine Wynne knew that with her progressing cancer, she would never again see the Sisters going on the new mission. With the Baltimore foundation only four years old, she parted with four of her dearest Sisters and two postulants. However, in deep faith, she felt that God would bless the community for the sacrifice by sending new members. Indeed it happened, but the price was painful. The separation scene was poignant for all and would long be remembered in the minds of those six: Sisters DeSales Browne, Vincent Browne, Stephana Warde, Sister Ignatius Sumner (lent until the group got established) and two aspirants, Kate Reynolds and Mary Maddigan.

Catherine Wynne died within a year. Her last duty was to change the Washington Infirmary into a Military Hospital. The medical faculty gave it to the military but insisted on the Sisters remaining in charge.

While Sister Ignatius and her five companions were traveling all over Mississippi and Alabama with the Confederates, her peers were nursing hundreds of sick and wounded of both armies. Terrible battles were fought along the Potomac and in the nearby states of Virginia, Maryland, and Pennsylvania.

The day of Catherine Wynne's interment, the Washington Infirmary burned. Three Sisters risked their lives trying to get patients out of the burning building. The hospital was relocated and renamed Douglas Hospital. Sister Ignatius' dear friend and contemporary, Sister Alphonsus, assumed leadership of the community in place of Catherine Wynne. Her friend, Sister Colette O'Conner, became administrator of the hospital. Twenty-two Sisters nursed there during the war. Sister Colette died on duty in 1864. At the demand of the soldiers, she was buried with full military honors and the rank of a major.

Catherine Wynne's legacy was in the women of faith and courage she left behind: "the small but noble band of self-sacrificing women consecrated to the highest ideals."[24]

To far away Mississippi, Sister Ignatius and the group came in 1860. Ten days after arrival, the school opened and was named St. Catherine's after Mother Catherine Wynne. Sister Ignatius taught advanced English classes and presided over the Music Department. In May, the second year of school, a naval bombardment began, and life as itinerant nurses was under way as described in her journal: "From Vicksburg to Jackson to Oxford to Canton, back to Jackson, then on to Meridian, to Shelby Springs, Alabama, then back and forth in 1864 negotiating with General Henry Slocum, Union Commander, to get the Sisters' property back from the Federals."

During this time, she kept the little money the Sisters had and negotiated charitably but astutely for provisions. The Confederate government never gave them any remuneration other than rations. Her tone is charitable, but she is astute in judging character or the lack thereof. Her chronicle is anecdotal and swift. She records scanty food. The callow officer's swagger, crude male nurses jumping into cots to play victims and receive food, bartering for eggs from a camp follower — all come to life in her descriptions and snatches of dialogue. Her devotion to wounded soldiers was unflagging whether Union or Confederate. Her faithfulness to transcribing even when weary, was admirable. While transporting the over 900 wounded from Jackson to Shelby Springs, they were attacked, on one occasion, by wildcats smelling blood. Etched in granite in Shelby Springs on a monument is a quatrain from her original poem composed while reflecting on death, an ever present reality in her life:

> *The silent dead, the silent dead*
> *I've lingered where they sleep in peace*
> *Where care, and want, or thought of dread*
> *There anguished vigils cease.*[25]

After the war, the Baltimore community for the second time tried to get her to return, but she begged to remain during Reconstruction.

After the war she used her connections in the North to network further to secure places for the education of many daughters of families who had lost everything during the war. She even accompanied some of the young ladies to flourishing academies where they received comparable college educations.[26]

Her obituary states: "Many of the young business men of this city will in memory go back to their early school days when she was their patient teacher."[27] This is a tribute to her ability to see a need and answer it by teaching at night young men who had to work in the day.

Sister Ignatius was the assistant to Sister DeSales, founder of the Vicksburg community, and convent treasurer. It was Sister Ignatius who was determined to build a first-class auditorium and academy and went to Chicago to see the best and most efficient buildings which might serve as models to imitate. In her tactful, charming manner, she defied the clergy and saw that a magnificent, efficient, and aesthetically pleasing building was raised, although it was much more expensive than that sanctioned by the hierarchy. Since she basically raised the money, she got by with it. She continued to teach the young ladies by day and at night school in the evenings. In later years, her sight failed her, but her mind was so well-trained and stored with knowledge she continued classes in reading, history, and math.[28]

At the end of the journal, she writes a note to Sister DeSales say-ing, "Please keep these manuscripts for us after you have finished with them, as all the latter part is from memory, and we have no other Record than this, which may be interesting to our Sisters at some future time if preserved." Someone took 11 pages of the manuscript and failed to return them. So when Sister's eyes had failed she dictated her memories to Sis-ter Angela Fedou who transcribed them. There was a lack of chronology in the original which was clarified in the enriched expanded journal. Placing a capital letter on "Record" shows how important this was to her. She must have emphasized to the young Sisters this importance of keeping a written record for posterity, since Sister Angela Fedou kept a very well-documented, meticulous diary of the Yellow Fever epidemic in Edwards, Mississippi, in 1897; the Sisters served there for a year. Sister Marcelline Street kept a less detailed, but equally interesting diary of the Sisters' mission with the Choctaws in Tucker, Mississippi, from 1885 until 1903 when the government relocated members of the tribe to Oklahoma.[29]

The headlines of the daily paper provide an appropriate summary of Sister Ignatius' life:

Sister Mary Ignatius had love, charity
entire life was devoted to the highest ideals[30]

Register Of The Events From The Foundation Of The Convent Of The Sisters Of Mercy, Vicksburg, Mississippi c. 1828 - 1895

The community of the Sisters of Mercy sent from Pittsburgh had been established for six years in Baltimore, under the Superiority of Mother Catherine Wynne,[1] in St. Peter's Parish, Reverend Edward Mc-Colgan pastor. Having taken the place of the Sisters of Charity, who had previously a school in the same locality, they experienced the effects of prejudice and other difficulties. The property had been presented to the Sisters of Mercy by Mrs. Emily McTavish, a granddaughter of Charles Carroll, of Carrollton; who with her sisters, Lady Wellesly, Lady Stafford and Duchess of Leeds, made many gifts of houses and lands to Religious Orders in their native country.[2]

Subservient to it was the public Infirmary, Washington, D.C.[3,] which was in a flourishing condition, even though up to 1860, only twenty members, most of them Novices, formed the Baltimore Community.[4] Death, which in a few years made such rapid havoc, including two of the most promising members in rapid succession, began already to cast his shadow in the Novitiate. Several applications...[had] been made to obtain new foundations but laborers were too few, and it was only...when Bishop Elder of Natchez[5] applied, warmly seconded by the Most Rev. Archbishop of Baltimore, Francis P. Kenrick, Bishop Elder assuring Rev. Mother that God would rapidly fill her Novitiate, that she consented to part with her Sisters. The Bishop's prophecy was fulfilled; subjects entered in rapid succession even though death thrust in his sickle.

[1]Mother Catherine Wynne was the third to join the Sisters of Mercy in the United States. She entered in 1844 in Pittsburgh. She started the foundation in Loretto, Pennsylvania, and established Baltimore in 1855 with only three companions and scarely any temporal means of support. She laid a firm foundation for the Sisters of Mercy by training young Sisters who would be outstanding Mercy leaders. (See Ignatius biography)

[2]McTavish, a Baltimore property owner, presented the residence adjoining the church to the Sisters and later a house for working girls. The Austin Carroll Annals say, "the house contained no furniture, poverty everywhere, Mother Catherine wondered from whence the furniture and next meal would come."

[3]Teaching hospital staffed by the Pittsburgh Sisters of Mercy, one of whose brothers was a doctor on the staff.

[4]Of the twenty members, four professed Sisters and two aspirants went to Vicksburg. By the end of the war there were 22 Sisters who had served in the hospital.

[5]Bishop William Henry Elder, Third Bishop of the Diocese of Natchez. A native of Maryland, Elder governed the Natchez Diocese from 1857-1880. He traveled his diocese on horseback and kept his own journal. His life parallels this journal and goes beyond. In 1880 he became Archbishop of Cincinnati. He returned in 1898 for Sister DeSales jubilee.

The Pastor of Vicksburg, Rev. Francis Xavier Leray, accompanied the little Foundation from Baltimore on October 9, 1860. Sister M. De-Sales Browne was Superioress; and the others were Sister M. Ignatius Sumner; Sister M. Vincent Browne; Sister Stephana Warde, lay Sister, and two postulants.[6]

How great was the anguish of separation, the same pangs of grief which had been often endured before by those who, for the salvation of souls, bid adieu to the dear nursery of their first religious days, where they have been so closely united to the religious companions of their sacrifices, and their devotions. The cry of Mother Catherine Wynne seems to resound even now in our ears as with anguish she repeated "O, I shall never see you more!" She was a devoted Religious, and strict disciplinarian and suffered much anxiety in the early struggles of the Community, which no doubt tended to develop the cancer, which had been twice operated on, and of which she died the year after our departure.

We parted that bright October evening full of sorrow, but full also of zeal for the salvation of souls; and after traveling[7] night and day through the beautiful scenery of our country, swiftly passing the winding course of rapid rivers; and mountains, standing like giant protectors over nestling towns, and villages at their base; forests with their magnificent foliage of Autumn leaves, until we came to the fields of mimic snow of the South,[8] bursting from green enclosures, as if to seek the sunshine.

Arriving in Vicksburg at 7 o'clock in the evening, we found Mr. Antonio Genella[9] and Clement Guidici with carriages awaiting us and cordial welcome. We were driven to Mr. Genella's house, where at the head of the stairs, stood the buoyant little figure of his wife, who welcomed us warmly from a heart full of affectionate cordiality. The light, glow, comfort and warmth of the surroundings astonished some of the Sisters, who had an idea that they were coming to some half Indian place, which would call forth all their fortitude as Missionaries[10] and had been mentally resolving to suffer all the imaginary deprivations patiently. We remained guests of Mr. Genella until Oct. 15, Feast of St. Theresa, when we took possession of the house designed for our Convent, beautifully situated on Crawford St. On Oct. 19 the Convent was blessed by the pastor and placed under the patronage of St. Catherine of Siena in memory of Rev. Mother Catherine of Baltimore, who from a small and comparatively recent establishment, had given four subjects[11]

[6]Agnes Maddigan and Kate Reynolds. Rose Farmer came a few months later, entering at Vicksburg on Feb. 7, 1861.

[7]The Sisters traveled by rail.

[8]Cotton in full bloom in October.

[9]Antonio Genella came from Switzerland; he had one of the largest mercantile houses in Vicksburg.

[10]The Sisters do go to the Choctaw Indians in Neshoba County later in 1885 and serve there until 1903, when the Government sent the Indians to reservations in Oklahoma.

[11]The four professed Sisters and 2 aspirants.

to the new foundation. Bishop Elder arrived in Vicksburg[12] on the 20th, giving the Sisters a cordial welcome; and on the 22nd, he presided at the opening of the school, delivering an eloquent address to the parents and children assembled.

There were about sixty children of both sexes at the opening, and the number soon increased to more than a hundred. Many of them had not had the advantage of religious training, but the soil of their hearts was fertile, and yielded readily to cultivation.[13] They improved rapidly in virtue and knowledge, and on Ascension day, the 9th of May, 1861, twenty three of them, ten boys and thirteen girls, made their first Holy Communion, after a retreat of three days and frequent, earnest exhortations from the Pastor.[14] They gave evident signs of fervor, and breakfasted afterwards at the Convent, spending the entire day on the grounds. On the 31st of the same month, a Sodality of the "Children of Mary," under the protection of Our Lady of Mercy, was instituted; twenty-two girls received the badge and Medal as candidates.[15]

Rose Farmer, of Baltimore, entered on the 7th of February, 1861, and was received with Mary Maddigan, in St. Paul's Church, by Bishop Elder on the 8th of April, the one as Sister M. Philomena, the other Sister M. Agnes.[16] Martha Newman of Vicksburg entered on the 2nd of March and Bessie Bury, of St. Louis, on the 25th of March.

On the 2nd of July, Feast of the Visitation, Kate Reynolds, one of the Baltimore postulants, was received, as lay Sister,[17] by Reverend Francis Xavier Leray, called in religion Sister M. Gertrude.[18] On the 1st of May, Mrs. Ann Pitcher, of New Orleans, offered to place at the disposal of the Sisters $1000, free of interest, for the purpose of building an addition to the Convent, but the offer could not be availed of, on account of the Civil War, which burst upon our peaceful little Convent like a thunderbolt. The Bishop added $2000, (loaned to us).

[12]From Natchez, 70 miles down river.

[13]The Expanded Journal says "they were from homes where dissipation and vice reigned." The neighbors complained of shanty Irish children; Father LeRay had to calm their fears. Visitation of families on the levee started immediately. The new immigrants were government employed in the '50s to build levees for flood control. The living conditions were squalid.

[14]Children, before 1911, did not receive Communion until they were in their teens.

[15]Group dedicated to devotion to Mary, meditation on Scripture, and works of mercy. In Vicksburg they attended funerals and different church liturgies after marching in procession three blocks from the school to the church.

[16]They received the habit after six months postulancy, where they had been dressed simply in black. A year of novitiate was required before final vows. It was a time for prayer, personal and communal, scripture study, learning the history, customs, charism of the Order. (see biographies)

[17]A lay Sister works in activities other than the academic programs, i.e., visitation of sick and culinary duties, freeing those in academic work from excessive domestic chores.

[18]Later Kate Reynolds, Sister Gertrude, was dismissed; Bessie Bury returned of her own accord to St. Louis because of ill health.

On the 19th of June, a distribution of Premiums took place, the number distributed being sixty-five. The Exhibition was opened by a dialogue between two large girls, which was well and gracefully spoken, and followed by an amusing dialogue by boys, which elicited great applause. Two other pieces were also spoken by girls, and the whole concluded with a speech by a boy. As there was not sufficient room in the house, a stage was erected on the gallery, which was festooned by curtains. Opposite was a platform upon which were the Rev. Mother, Reverend F. X. Leray, Reverend P. LeCorre[19] and Reverend Father Elia[20], also Mayor [R. H.] Crump, who gave the Premiums.[21] The two highest were awarded to Julia Condon and William Rohrbacker, for Excellence.

The Mayor delivered an appropriate and encouraging address to all assembled, and Father Leray concluded the whole by suitable advice to the children.

The first retreat for the renovation of vows had been given at the usual time, by Bishop Elder. The annual retreat[22] was now given between 20th and 25th of August, by Reverend Father Smulders, C.S.S.R.,[23] who had already given three retreats to the Baltimore Community. School reopened on the 1st Monday of September with 55 boys and 87 girls. For Sunday school 78 boys and 121 girls with about 25 Negroes. On the 5th of September, Martha Newman and Bessie Bury received the white veil from Father Leray, in St. Paul's Church, taking the names of Sisters M. Teresa and M. Josephine. Father Leray gave us the retreat for the renovation of vows with much unction and earnestness. Twelve girls of the B.V.M. Sodality received the white ribbon of Profession on Sunday, the 8th of December walking down to the church in procession, with veils and wreaths and lighted candles; where, after an impressive discourse from Father Leray, one of the girls read the Act of Profession, and they were invested with the ribbon and Medal.

War, having been declared in 1861, in the May following, of 1862, the Northerners came with their gun boats to attack Vicksburg, and commenced to shell the place; our school was gradually broken up; by the second week in ... same month, all the inhabitants having fled into the surrounding country; those who could not get houses camping out in the woods, and living in caves which they dug in the sides of the

---

[19]Paul Marie Lacorre, native of France, pastor of Yazoo City from 1856.

[20]Basilio Elia, young priest. In 1861 he served Catholics in North Mississippi. He died in 1863 from overexhaustion ministering to Union soldiers wounded in Vicksburg and serving as chaplain to Holy Cross Sisters on the hospital boat "Red Rover."

[21]Some type of award; in later years medals cut by local jewelers.

[22]The Sisters of Mercy traditionally observed a three-day retreat the last three days of the year and renewed vows together the last day of December or around the first of January. They traditionally had an eight-day retreat in the summer. Conferences and meditations usually were given by a religious-order priest.

[23]A religious-order Redemptorist priest.

hills.[24] On Ascension day, Father Leray, being anxious about our safety, six of the sisters accepted the invitation of Major Cook and his wife, went to their plantation[25] and four of them remained a month,[26] three of them having returned to the convent to nurse the sick soldiers, with which the house was filled after their departure. Sickness, terror, death, reigned everywhere. Soldiers without shelter, or else lying on the bare floor, were scattered through the town.[27] Finally, a Government Hospital was established at Mississippi Springs[28] and the Sisters were solicited to preside.

On the 17th of June, two of the sisters and a postulant came out to prepare the house, the rest following on Corpus Christi. About 400 soldiers arrived in the course of a week, and in two weeks we had 700. The sick had been hurried out of Vicksburg, due to fear it would be taken by the enemy. The house was dirty and neglected, entirely unfurnished, the mattresses burned on the cars[29] coming out, and [we] were without the necessary means of cooking, or supplying the soldiers with necessities, so that the Sisters suffered much in seeing the sick suffer. It was not until the latter part of July that the serious shelling of Vicksburg by the enemy commenced.[30] The government having concluded, after much vacillating, to break up the hospital at Mississippi Springs, as being too remote from the cars for the sick, the Sisters were solicited by the surgeon in charge to accompany him to the Institute for the Deaf and Dumb in Jackson, Mississippi, which had been taken as a hospital. Some of the Sisters went to assist in cleaning the house, and we were finally settled there on the "Feast of All Saints." [November 1]

[24]City was shelled off and on for over a year. The naval bombardment lasted from May 19, 1862, until July 24, 1862. The Federals' gunboats periodically shelled the city during the period February 2-May 3, 1863. The siege began May 19, 1863. Elder's diary records that two columns had been knocked down from the convent, a shell came through an upstairs room. The Church, on the other hand, had some nine holes through the walls and windows. Sunday morning in May Michael Donovan, local saloon keeper, had his arm shot off at the church door. Father Charles Heuze had his coattail shot to ribbons.

[25]"Hardtimes" in Bovina, 10 miles east of Vicksburg.

[26]The Sisters took as much chapel furniture as they could move to the Cooks. They instructed the Blacks belonging to the Cook family in Catholic doctrine and to some from the neighboring plantations.

[27]Many died from measles and typhoid fever. Many died in the convent and school. The records of these deaths are at the old Court House Museum.

[28]Mississippi Springs was between Clinton and Raymond, closest to Clinton, 30 miles east of Vicksburg near Cooper's Well. The Hubert Spengler family owned the property but sold it to the Joe Dehmer family who presently own it.

[29]Railroad cars — the only transportation.

[30]In the opening months of the war, Kate Reynolds was advised to return home, which she did on June 21, 1863.

After being there a week, finding the surgeon perfectly equal to the task of the whole management of the house, which contained only about three hundred sick, the Sisters went where their services were much more needed, taking charge of an hospital at Oxford, Mississippi [31] on the "Feast of the Presentation of the Blessed Virgin." [February 2, 1863]

Some of the Sisters were detained in Jackson, until they could hear whether it was desirable to join the others, which they did in a few days. They were treated with much kindness by Mr. Angelo Miazza,[32] where they stayed, and by Father Orlandi.[33] Father Leray accompanied us. The hospital at Oxford was composed of twelve large buildings, forming an immense circle.[34] It had been used as a college, and contained about one thousand sick.[35] Many were extremely ill and neglected and the whole place was in a disorderly condition. Here, as we ate our corn bread without salt and drank our sage tea, or sweet potato coffee, according to taste, Reverend Mother read us our morning lecture,[36] as the distance to the various wards was so great that we could only return at meal time. A good woman one day brought us some eggs and butter from the country, which we considered a great boon, and when we succeeded in getting some apples to cook for the sick, they seemed as precious as gold. In all our hospital campaign, Rev. Mother prepared the delicacies for the sick, her experience and her thoughtfulness were of incalculable value.[37] It was a wide field of labor and the place, and the condition of the sick, were gradually improving and even the invariable collegiate tobacco juice, was disappearing from the walls, when, at the end of the month, we were warned to prepare in haste for flight, as the Federals were momentarily expected. All of the sick who could be moved were

---

[31]University of Mississippi Campus.

[32]Angelo Miazza, an Italian immigrant and pioneer businessman; he operated a first-class boarding house near the State Capitol. His descendants became city leaders and his granddaughter became a Sister of Mercy, Sister Mary Vincent. The Jackson Daily paper May 15, 1875 advertised "Angelo Miazza Bar and Restaurant. Elegant sleeping rooms $2.00 per night."

[33]Francis Orlandi, Italian priest and Jackson pastor. After serving in Jackson with the Sisters, he returned to Italy totally disheartened after having the Jackson church and two makeshift chapels destroyed by the three Federal occupations.

[34]The Sisters nursed at the Barnard Observatory. The 12 buildings of the University are much the same (see picture).

[35]From Battles of Shiloh and Corinth. Shiloh, Apr. 6 & 7, 1862 — one of the most violent battles of the war, killed or wounded Union 13,047, Confederates 10,699. Corinth: Union 2,520, Confederates 4,233. Shiloh foreshadowed the loss of Memphis and the Memphis and Charleston Railroad from Memphis to east of Corinth. Ironically, the Mercy Sisters from Cincinnati came on a hospital ship down the Tennessee River and took the Union wounded back to Cincinnati from the Battle of Shiloh.

[36]Reading from Scripture, Lives of the Saints.

[37]It is here recorded in the "Expanded Journal" that Sister DeSales put the Sisters to bed, washed their coifs and guimps, spent the greater part of the night gathering wood and keeping up the fire, while the Sisters slept.

hurried off; about sixty of the most ill being left.[38] After an uncertainty of two days, we started in box cars, and two hours after we left, the Federals so took possession of Oxford. We passed the night on some mattresses, grateful to be so comfortably lodged. We arrived in Canton, Miss. the evening of the next day. The guard at the depot, catching a glimpse of our coifs,[39] hastened towards us, thinking we were wounded Yankees and was somewhat abashed to find only peaceful Sisters. He asked Father Leray if we were all his daughters, and said, glancing at the black habit, "Poor things! I suppose their Mother is dead." Our cheery host of the hotel welcomed us warmly in a primitive way. "You are welcome, my girls, to the parlor; all the rest of the house is full." He bade us farewell the next morning with the same original epithet, which, however, did not seem disrespectful in his mouth. The hotel being crowded, we got some comforts and passed the night on the parlor floor, in company with four servant girls who were with us, these girls[40] having joined us at Oxford, where we were at first almost without assistance.

The following morning at 10 o'clock we arrived in Jackson and went to Father Orlandi's house, everywhere assisted and protected by Father Leray. We remained at Father Orlandi's two weeks attending to his house, supplied with rations by the government and occupying ourselves with his church.[41] There was an alarm of fire one night and danger of the church, when Father Orlandi in his agitation, climbed to the roof with a small watering pot to extinguish the fire, which made us all laugh, though otherwise not amusing to watch a fire in the front yard, on a December night. We had begun to feel very anxious about hospital work, when Doctor Warren Brickell, of New Orleans, who had taken a large house, called the "Dixon House," in Jackson, invited us through Father Leray to assist him. Accordingly, we took possession of a little cottage of four rooms, and as our man "Dick" and some of the girls who came from Vicksburg still remained with us, we commenced our work on Christmas Eve. Some of the officers would have preferred having the management themselves, as, here, as elsewhere, there was less opportunity for private speculations at the sacrifice of the comfort of the sick, when the Sisters were on duty, so that the Doctor allowed himself to be influenced for a time, until receiving a better acquaintance with the true state of things. We had a chapel, community room, and two bed rooms, and in our little Chapel diligently fixed up, Father Leray gave us our three days' retreat which gave us fresh courage.

---

[38]940 evacuated.

[39]White cloth flowing around the face covering the hair.

[40]High school girls and older women who came to work with the Sisters referred to sometimes as domestics.

[41]At that time, the church bells had been given at request of General John C. Pemberton to be melted down for shells. The bells rang three times a day and were warnings of fire, etc.

The Steward, a smart, but unprincipled fellow, who had been with us at the other hospitals, followed us here also, and continued his aggrandizement until the Doctor discovered his doings. On our flight from Oxford, as we were vainly trying to rest, while a broom handle stuck in the side of one, another half smothered by a mattress thrown on her, and a third disputed possession of a comfort with the insect, relics, too often the companions of soldiers. The soldiers crowded on the top of the cars, a dangerous proceeding, but Tom, the steward, soon put them to flight from ours, by poking out his head and gravely asking them, "if they had had the smallpox, as there was a case inside." Our hospital arrangements began to improve, an additional house was taken, and a ward for the wounded erected. Ladies came occasionally and bestowed niceties on the sick, though most kindness was extended to other hospitals.

Some Baptisms took place; one poor fellow died immediately after its being administered; a wounded officer was brought in, in a desperate condition; he asked Sister himself for baptism, and died shortly after. Several sick prisoners were brought in. One, a boy of 16 years of age, full of spirit, naturally included us among his enemies and was curt enough, until he was convinced nothing but kindness was meant him; he was too young to brave the rigors of war and soon died, and the [male] nurse said to the other prisoners, "Now, you see that he is buried like our own men; he has been treated like them." Indeed, we were glad to see that there were great good feelings towards each other on both sides. Another prisoner, dying of pneumonia, expressed a great desire to see the men of his company; Sister asked the Surgeon, who sent to prison for them. About dusk, several came in their blue uniforms, followed by their guard, in Gray, bearing a flaming torch which threw picturesque light on the group around the bed. Sister asked the dying man if he knew them, and a smile of pleasure lighted up his face, as he called their names and pressed their hands; in a moment he said, "Where are you? I cannot see," and the prisoner was free at last, the guard with his flambeau[42] wishing they had all gone the same way. The affection which members of the same Company had for each other was remarkable and truly fraternal. About this time, Pat, a little guard of our own, was taken sick, and the Doctor asked him, "if he got his medicine." "Yis Docther," he said, "but it wouldn't sthop wid one." (it was an emetic).[43] The Doctor laughed very heartily. The same little fellow always kept a jealous eye on his provender,[44] even if he could not eat it, and if any one came near the eatables on his chair, would call out, "Hould!" in a warning voice.

The Doctor did not know why another man did not get better. Sister said, "I expect you have been eating molasses;[45] the man declared he had not. Sister said, "Don't I see it on you face;" he then wiped his mouth,

[42]Flaming torch.

[43]Causes one to vomit. Common medicine for almost anything.

[44]Food, probably grain and corn and oats.

[45]Molasses gives diarrhea, diluted used as stool softener among babies, harsh laxative among adults.

and said, "I only eat a few."[46] The Doctor was amused at the ruse, to discover the truth. On the 4th of July, 1863, Vicksburg was surrendered to Genl. Grant, to the astonishment of a people who believed the war would be interminable; but want of care, provisions and clothing did the work of demoralization.[47] Grant attacked Jackson; fighting continued for some days, and cannon were planted near our hospital, but afterwards removed.[48] The wounded were brought in, one of them with his fingers shot off, and his leg torn by a shell. He suffered terribly and died saying, "Tell my brother to avenge my death!" Another had the artery of his neck severed, and it was necessary to sit by him all the time, with the thumb pressed on it. He was from Tennessee and got his idea of Catholics from bad books and bad preaching, and therefore would not let a Sister come near him; finally he yielded and was never satisfied without one. Another, who had been brought from another hospital, with his blister grown into his side, turned with indignation from the offer of a Sister to dress it. When she came for the third time with milk and water to dress it and told him, if she did not do it, the Doctor would come around and tear it off, he burst into tears, and asked her to forgive him, that he had been taught to believe badly of Sisters. Many other poor fellows not well cared for in other hospitals, were brought to us, but some were too far gone to recruit.[49]

Jackson surrendered[50] and Johnson's army evacuated the place.[51] The Federals came in, and fires sprung up, at the given sound of a trumpet. On pretense of burning some barrels of pitch, the Catholic church was set on fire, the Irish companies having been marched out of town previously. A physician on Grant's Grand Staff did his best to save the church;[52] he was a fervent Convert, but all in vain; the officers,

---

[46]Colloquial way country people referred to grits and molasses as some grits some molasses; few grits few molasses.

[47]Citizens knew the importance of Vicksburg. In Union hands the River transportation could be blocked and in a matter of time the War would be lost. Citizens held out eating dogs and rats — printing news on wallpaper.

[48]On May 14 Union forces led by General Grant entered Jackson after a sharp fight, and on the 16th Sherman's XV Corps, after wrecking the railroad and destroying much of the central city, but not the hospital, went on to Vicksburg. On July 10 Sherman's Columns returned to the Jackson area following the capture of Vicksburg July 4 and after several days of fierce skirmishing compelled the Confederates led by Genl. Joseph E. Johnston to evacuate Jackson on the night of July 16th. Jackson was known as Chimneyville, for miles only chimneys remained to indicate former sites of homes.

[49]Older meaning of the word in Webster dictionary, restore vigor or health.

[50]Sherman invested and shelled Jackson for 7 days. Union troops took all government stores. Sherman reported to Grant July 18, 1863, "Jackson will no longer be a point of danger."

[51]General Joseph E. Johnston's army vainly attempted to salvage the desperate situation at Vicksburg during the period May 13-July 4, 1863.

[52]Dr. H. S. Hewitt, a Catholic convert, his brother an associate of Father Isaac Hecker, founder of the Paulist Fathers. During occupation of Vicksburg he set up his office in St. Paul's church possibly to save its destruction.

while they sympathized with the citizens in words, ordered the hose to be cut, so that no water could reach the flames and when Father Leray, observed it, he was insulted, on which he replied, "You would not dare to insult me, but that you know my office prevents resentment." Father Leray then bore the B[blessed] Sacrament to our little Chapel, the tears streaming from his eyes. The Doctor was so horrified at this, and other outrages, that he resigned his appointment. Some of the soldiers, who came to get religious objects, evidently did not know which side was right; they had been prevailed upon to enter the Army on their arrival in the country. The substitutes for the church were twice afterwards destroyed and desecrated by the same Army.[53] Some gentlemen asked an Irish woman, what was the reason the Catholic churches were destroyed, and not the Protestant? She quickly replied, "When the Divil sends his immissaries, sure he always take care of his own." As all government stores were now taken possession of by the Federals, we began to suffer the want of many things. We did, however the best we could, for Father Leray, who observed with a smile "that we must have been hard pushed, for he had the heel of a loaf for three days." One of our sick men was so terrified at the roar of the cannon,[54] which he had never heard before, that after walking up and down stupefied, with his hat on, John departed, without leave, for some Utopia where guns were not. Another who had been ordered to Brookhaven, said "he would not go to Brookhaven, Workhaven, or any other haven," so he departed for Vicksburg where he enjoyed peace under the Stars and Stripes. Some were all on fire, and would have defied a whole army single handed. Our position being dangerous from lawless soldiery, a Federal guard was appointed for the hospital. We observed how completely a man was transformed by war. One who, when sick a few days before, had been cowardly as Caesar was, now returned from battle, with eyes luminous and distended, and so wholly transformed, one could imagine that a hero of Homer's, a Ulysses, Agamemnon, a Hector stood before them. The influence of religion was also sometimes striking even when they did not understand it. A fine young South Carolinian Captain, being brought in ill, was out of his mind and swore continually except when a Sister came in, and was generally controlled by them though his ravings were of the ballroom. He would only take his medicine from Reverend Mother, whom he imagined his "Aunt Margaret!" The Georgians we had were true-hearted, and the Texans, though wild, were faithful. "Look,

[53]While the siege was going on in Vicksburg, the Jackson congregation fixed up the largest hall remaining in town for church. One week after Mass was celebrated, Sherman's army was back. It was deliberately ransacked, altar crucifix broken, vessels stolen. A chalice was returned by a Union Catholic soldier.

[54]The hospital was hit during the 7-day bombardment, but the shell passed through the ward without exploding.

Sister," said one, "See what Texas does for the Confederacy," pointing from a window to a long line of lean travel-worn cattle. His glands had suppurated[55] and he died a few minutes after.

When the bombardment of Jackson commenced, all escaped who could; a part of a shell fell into the wounded ward and took off the corner of the house and exploded in the chicken coop. The cook who was very fat, like the ostrich, stuck her head under the steps, leaving a large surface of body exposed to danger, her sister, who was indignant at her for some sauciness, poked at her, posteriorly, with a large fork, and she escaped with the enemy in the rear. Father Leray made his Will, and said Mass at 4 o'clock, the shelling having already commenced. The Sisters assisted at it, feeling every moment would be their last. After Mass we went through the now deserted streets, and spent the day in the State House, being less in the line of attack. There we spent an anxious day, and the next day were ordered to pack, which we did hastily, and followed the Army across the Pearl River.[56] Doctor Furniss, faithful and true, hurrying back to get some of our coifs and gamps (sic),[57] hanging on a line. Dick proved faithless and left us. Our bonnets were destroyed by the soldiers, and our books and other articles carried off.[58] We spent the night in a cottage, on the floor or leaning on our baggage, there being but one bed where we could take a nap in turn. A Sister, being told to go to bed, and after the closest reconnoitering, finding none, concluded the ghost of one would satisfy her conscientious scruples on the subject of obedience, laid down on the floor, surrounded by the post and frame of a dismantled bed-stead, and comical enough she looked, when the rest hunted her up. On July 16th, we set out again in boxcars. We set out on a journey of discovery. We stopped at Meridian, where a polite darkey offered us the hospitality of his Mistress' house, but before we could find out where she lived, the cars moved on a little, and the man did not reappear. We boiled coffee on the roadside and Doctor Warren Brickell's man, Horace, would come and get some for him.

We stopped next at Demopolis, for a night and day,[59] and then like poor "Joe," we kept moving on. And next stopping at the hotel in Selma, where we found a Vicksburg neighbor; thence proceeding 60 miles,

---

[55]Expanded with puss; came to a head.

[56]They stayed in the State House two or three days and heard Mass in the chapel of the hospital; at 4:00 a.m. Johnston ordered the Confederates to retreat beyond the Pearl River as far as Meridian; the Sisters accompanied the refugee train with wounded.

[57]Coif, the white cloth around the face; guimpe, long circular white collar from neck to waist.

[58]Bishop Elder arrived in Jackson soon afterwards. He recorded in his diary "I could not talk much, I felt myself choked with sadness and indignation. All the stores are broken open and sacked. The soldiers were carrying off boxes that seem to contain books of the State House Library. One fourth of the town is in ashes." The makeshift chapel was ransacked. Two large statues smashed and the altar used as a butcher's block.

[59]The Sisters slept in a deserted house.

above, we stopped at a Watering Place called, "Shelby Springs," which the Doctor selected, as the most suitable place for a hospital,[60] much to the chagrin of the "Refugees,"[61] who thought they had secured a pleasant abode for the sumner.

The main building was in two parts, and a line of cottages, open to every wind of heaven, extended to a considerable distance. The ball-room was converted into a Surgical Ward. We had found whole rations, but not too much. We were now put on half rations until the sick came, the dirt, being as usual, in melancholy ascendancy, and one of the Sisters, not yet recovered from the jaundice, from exposure. We had refused all compensation from the beginning, but fortunately we had a little money left to buy what provisions we could find.[62] A sharp old Hoosier woman used to come sometimes to drive hard bargains; she much desired the pattern of our capes. Gradually the place was put in order and patients came in. One good old soldier, who looked like an old Mother, and indeed had been so to his brothers and sisters, was helping Sister by washing a hearth, in one of the cottages, when a jaunty, airish [sic] fellow of his own company, who was sick in the same room, said: "Is it pops'ble [sic] you are brought down so low?" The old fellow answered (scrubbing away with undaunted energy), "Them that this war don't bring down aint bringable," an unanswerable reply to the would-be hero. The old

[60]Sixty miles northeast of Selma. A hotel with mineral waters being used as a recruitment and training center by the Confederates when the war began. A former spa converted into a hospital — a retreat and convalescent home for soldiers until they could return to duty or were given leave. It was on the railroad, had a good water supply, and was remote from scenes of battle, three requisites for hospitals. Its location in a valley made it somewhat damp.
A further description from a love letter from James Wilson Moore to Alice Petrie of Jackson, August 11, 1863, Shelby Springs, Alabama:
"Miss Alice,
I cannot tell you how very sorry I was to leave Jackson without seeing you. If it had been possible I should have gone out to bid you 'good bye', but we rec'd orders to move very unexpectedly and just at dark, and I was forced to submit to the disappointment. We at first rec'd orders to move our hospital to Lauderdale Springs, Miss., but when we arrived at Meridian, we found orders awaiting us to go on to Shelby Springs, Alabama, so we came on to this place and took possession. We found a very gay and fashionable crowd here, enjoying themselves to their hearts' content at this pleasant place among the mountains; but great was their consternation and disappointment when it was made known to them that their sojourn here was at an end. I wish you could have been here to witness the wonder that was excited by our arrival. The eight Sisters of Mercy with their priest who arrived now to care with us, caused no small amount of staring & whispering by the vistors (among the ladies, of course). There were a number of ladies here from Mississippi, refugees, and I feel very sorry that we had to break up their summer residence here.
This is a very pleasant place and an excellent locality for a hospital. It is immediately on the Ala. & Tenn. Rivers R.R., about 65 miles from Selma. The Springs are in a cool, pleasant, shady valley among the mountains, in a part of the country that has not yet felt the desolating effect of this terrible war. The water is very fine, five bold gushing springs (sulphur free, Stone & Chalybeate) within one area of less than an hundred yards in diameter. We have a hospital capacity for three hundred patients, and very comfortable quarters for ourselves...."

[61]Loyal Confederate Creole families from New Orleans who were exiled by the Federals. General Benjamin Butler made them take a loyalty oath and made life miserable for them. Amanaide Poursine's family was among them. Amanaide was later received when the Sisters returned to Vicksburg.

[62]The Sisters never took salary but were always permitted to draw Army rations.

man was so attached to us, that when ordered to his command, tears ran down his face, while he looked at us, and held his untasted dinner before him.

There was a funny, dumpy, old nurse, who, when Sister asked him every day for fun, how many he wanted dinner for, always said: "Twinty one — there's Brough and meself, and man in blue begant," & throughout the whole list. To our great regret, Doctor Brickell was removed, and then followed several, whose whole care was self aggrandizement and neglect of duty, which example was followed by inferior officers, the sick suffering in consequence, and influenced, in many cases, to believe that they suffered through the Sisters' fault. Through representations made to the Medical Director, after sending a suitable person to ascertain the true state of the case, Doctor Brickell was returned, and though towards the close of the war there, was less provision in the Country, yet, all resources were made available, and the sick had better and more food, than they had had at any previous time. Doctor Brickell himself having made nothing off of the Confederacy, as he said, but a mosquito bar. We had the consolation of the return of some to the faith, who had been negligent, and the baptism of others, sick and dying, but the demoralizing effect of the war was such, that it was easier to die well, than to live well.[63]

Father Leray made Altar wine out of grapes squeezed in a tub, we sewed our own clothes with white thread, and we made him pants out of a shawl, and a brown delaine shirt from a dress. A calico for our postulant cost $113, and she was much afraid that Father would covet it, as a homespun dress had gone for a shirt. We had a Profession[64] here, and Mass, and all our religious exercises, except Office,[65] our labor and privations were made sweet, by the hope of reward to come. Our recreations[66] were always pleasant, Father Leray in the midst of us cheering

[63]Three times as many Confederate soldiers died from diseases as were killed in battle. The most common diseases were malaria, pneumonia, and dysentery. From one of the few surviving records of Shelby Springs hospital, patients were diagnosed as having a variety of other ailments including: "anemia, asthma, diarrhea chronica, erysipelas, febris continuens and remittens, gonorrhea, hepatitis, jaundice, neuralgia, pulmonalsis, rheumatic opthalmia, rubeola, scarbutus, spinal meningitis, syphilis and ulcus."

[64]Sister M. Teresa Newman, Jan. 6, 1864; she had entered in Vicksburg in 1860 and was from Warren County (Vicksburg) (See biography).

[65]The psalms three times a day — Matin, Lauds, Compline.

[66]Sisters would take one hour a day to be together, relax and call it recreation.

and sustaining. A remarkable instance occurred, of grace lost by one soul, given to another. A soldier who had been baptized Catholic, but had not practiced his religion, was receiving instructions, in order to prepare well for death, but the Methodist Minister, who continually visited the hospital distributing tracts, and talking to this man, captured his soul, and he would listen to no further instructions, but as he was dying, he whispered as Father Leray passed, "Glory!" and Father Leray replied: "I fear that won't save you." The man in the next bed said. "Father, I have listened to all you said and I believe in the Catholic Church and wish to be baptized." From time to time other souls were rescued and consoled in their last moments. Bishop [John] Quinlan, of Mobile, gave the Sisters a retreat, and also preached on the grounds, the soldiers crowding round to listen with attention. He refuted publicly one of the Methodist preachers, who had challenged him. Our Bishop Elder visited us and wished us to return home,[67] as the children needed our care. He thought it would be better to work to undertake our charge again. Accordingly, Father Grignon came in the last days of January, but not understanding the difficulties in the way, he had not secured passes, or anything; but the greatest opposition was manifested to the step by the surgeon in charge and the sick themselves. However, as one desired only to do the Will of God, two of the Sisters therefore went (as it was necessary to take many precautions for such a journey) on Jan. 29th to apply to Genl. Polk,[68] commander of the Division for permission and means to go to Vicksburg. His gentle, amiable wife obtained us an interview, and we stated our request, which he could not grant for some time, he said, on account of some military obstacle.[69] We were treated with the greatest kindess by Captain [J. J.] Fitzpatrick, Provost Marshal of Meridian, at the headquarters of the commander, also on our journey back to Shelby Springs.

　　　Father Mathurin Grignon had brought from Natchez, the only place from which we could receive letters from the North, the notice of the death of Sister M. Regina Browne,[70] Sister to two of the Members

---

[67]Bishop Elder was insistent that they return and resume as much normality as possible. There was little regard for property. Bishop Elder went to Vicksburg after the siege. He and Father Heuze went to General Grant to request protection for the Sisters' Convent and permission for them to reclaim it. Since Father Heuze was attending the Union soldiers without pay, Grant provided provisions, horse and buggy and forage for them. Grant directed the Bishop to Genl. James B. McPherson, who received him pleasantly and assured him the convent would be protected. A few days before the Sisters arrived, Gen. Henry Slocum had taken it over for staff officers quarters. On returning to Natchez, Bishop Elder had been banished from Union occupied Natchez for refusing to say public prayers for the U. S. government. Elder's Diary

[68]Lt. Gen. Leonidas Polk of the Dept. of Alabama, Mississippi and East Louisiana and first bishop of the Episcopal Diocese of Louisiana (1843 Thibodaux) prior to entry into the Confederate Army. He was a graduate of West Point, later killed in Georgia, Pine Mountain 1864, Sherman's March.

[69]Refused because of the danger — too much military movement in the area.

[70]Sister Regina second daughter of the Brownes, always delicate, remained in Baltimore, and labored at Douglas Hospital and the Washington prisons.

of our Community, making the loss of the Baltimore Community very severe, in the course of three years, four for our foundation, the Mother Superior[71] and two Sisters, by death from Cancer, another promising Member by Consumption, and another Sister of Rev. Mother DeSales, who joined the Community of Mercy in Buffalo,[72] Our Lord no doubt wishing to prove the fidelity of their present good and pious Superior, M. Alphonsus Atkinson.[73] On the 1st of the following July died Sister M. Colette,[74] Superior of a hospital in Washington, D.C., one of the Baltimore Community, and the last member of the Pittsburgh Community, who had composed the original foundation in Baltimore. Father Grignon pursued his journey home and the event justified the precautions we had taken, for a few days after, a Yankee raid which was then in progress took place, destroying the whole country from Vicksburg to beyond Meridian. Some time after, we received a letter from the Bishop, urging us to return as soon as the country was in a condition to travel.[75] Father applied again to Genl. Polk for passes, which he granted, but would give us no facility. In the meantime, he was ordered to the field, and Genl. Johnson[76] took his place, and granted us, upon application passes, transportation, and leave of absence for Father.[77] Accordingly, on the 23rd of May[1864] Rev. Mother, having, with the Bishop's cordial approbation, decided to leave four Sisters to take care of the sick,[78] we left them with sorrowful hearts, feeling the greatness of the sacrifice, and the uncertainty before us.[79]

We arrived in Selma that evening. The next evening saw us in Meridian, but about three miles before we reached that place, our car ran off the track, and turned over, saved from a deep pool of muddy water only by the trunk of a tree, which upheld us in falling by the will of

---

[71]Mother Catherine Wynne was the superior, Sisters Veronica and Regina Brown, both young Sisters, died at the Washington Infirmary and Sister Aloysius McCarthy, a young sister, made her vows on her deathbed.

[72]Teresa Browne, third daughter of the Brownes. She was first to enter in Buffalo, 1861, later became Mother M. Joseph Browne, died in 1917.

[73]Same age and same group as Sister Ignatius and Sister Vincent Browne; they had been young Sisters in Baltimore together. The group was small when the six left for Vicksburg (4 professed Sisters, 2 postulants).

[74]She died on duty, was buried with full military honors as a major by demand of the soldiers.

[75]Bishop Elder anticipated the difficulty of getting the property back from the Union occupation. Since his banishment, he had no influence and he feared permanent loss of the property. In the period — Feb. 3-March 6, 1864, General Sherman with a formidable force advanced from Vicksburg to Meridian and then returned to Vicksburg, cutting a swath of destruction across the state.

[76]General Joseph E. Johnston C.S.A.

[77]Father Leray did not stay with the Sisters all of the time. He was on the scene at the May 12, 1863 Battle of Raymond. (See Leray's biography)

[78]Sister M. Vincent was left in charge.

[79]Sister DeSales and Sister Ignatius made the journey May 23, 1864.

our good God and the Help of Christians, whose feast it was.[80] All were
unhurt, though frightened. The greatest kindness was shown by everyone to us. The rest of the way, a miscellaneous jumble of men, women,
trunks, soldiers and Sisters traversed in mud-cars. Father got permission, an unusual circumstance, for us to stay in the cars all night, from
the President of the road, though Captain and Mrs. [J. J.] Fitzpatrick
wanted us to stay there, but as it was more convenient for us to remain
where we were,[81] they brought us supplies and breakfast, most kindly.
Our travelling was every way facilitated by the respect and esteem felt
by everyone for Father Leray.

The next morning we started for Jackson, the railroad having been
completed the day before. We arrived safely in the evening in the neighborhood of [the] Pearl River, and taking a carriage, crossed the river on
a flat boat, and went to the house of Mrs. Lucy in Jackson.[82] The next
day was Corpus Christi, the sweetest Feast of the year, but on account
of some difficulty in opening the doors of the little place they had for a
church, and not expecting a priest, as their own had gone to Europe, we
were obligated to do without Mass. The Pastor of the place, discouraged
at having his little church three times destroyed, had gone to Italy.

On Friday, we started in an ambulance procured by Father from
Genl. Wirt Adams, with a Flag of Truce, accompanied by Captain Chamberlain, Genl. Pro. Marshal, whose acquaintance we had made in the
upset of the cars, and a private with the flag. We reached Messinger's
Ferry late that evening, having passed through a desolated, and destroyed region, everywhere, as far as Vicksburg, showing the marks of
relentless and savage destruction.[83]

After crossing the Ferry, we went up a little ascent, to the house
of Mrs. Messinger, who very hospitably offered us sleeping accommo-
dations. Provisions we had with us. It was a fine house, and had been
splendidly furnished, of which there still remained articles, but much
had been destroyed by the Federals. Her daughter, an agreeable young
married woman, gave us some excellent music, and some patriotic songs,
seeming to have the same ardent love of country, which the Southern

[80]Title of a feast day of Mary, the Mother of God.

[81]Probably stayed to guard the trunks.

[82]The Pearl River formed a natural boundary east of Jackson. The bridge had been destroyed by the
Union Army. J.W.K. Lucy family, Catholic. In 1860, Lucy was a city constable; in 1864 an alderman.

[83]In the hospitals the Sisters had seen what war did to human bodies; now they saw what it could do
to countryside and property.

women almost universally have. We slept comfortably that night and left refreshed the next morning, grateful for the kindness received. How our dear Lord takes care of his own under all circumstances.

The hills and hollows of the road became more numerous as we proceeded; here and there were the dead carcasses of animals, and numerous deserted encampments. We stopped at Mrs. Fox's about fifteen miles from Vicksburg; she gave us buttermilk and rolls. Tears came in her eyes as she looked at the dress (uniforms of our escort) and uttered, "God, bless that uniform." We reached Vicksburg at about 3 o'clock on the 28th of May and were detained at the lines, until word could be sent to Headquarters. In the meantime the gentlemen of our party conversed with the Federal Officers. We were detained an hour or so before word came back that the Sisters could come in, but no one else. We took leave of Father with heavy hearts, for all we had seen and heard looked unpromising for our future. Conducted, therefore, by a guard who led us on at a leisurely gait, talking to some women as he marched in front of us. When we arrived near the Court House, the voice of a profane Negro, who formerly lived near us, shouted out, cursing and talking of us to the black soldiers round him. This first salute gave us an idea of the difficulties the Negroes caused; however, they seemed well disposed to us, probably because we used to teach Negro Sunday school.[84]

We proceeded to Headquarters to obtain a pass for Father Leray to come in for a day or two. The Adjutant Genl., Col. Rogers, seemed to be willing to concede anything, when Genl. Slocum,[85] the officer in Command entered. He seemed not in a very good humor, and was agitated at the bear [sic] idea of letting in a Confederate Chaplain, to take the plan of the fortifications and flatly refused, demurring also at our taking out lunch to him and would not let us send anything to the Sisters.[86]

We saw the U. States Flag, waving at our Convent home opposite, and our hearts sank when we were told it had only been erected a few days before, and the house occupied for Military purposes. We were immediately shown to Mr. Genella's, still attended by our guard, who from first manifesting a rough curiosity, appeared to feel a growing interest.

After the first greetings had passed between ourselves and our old friends the Genella's, they hurriedly packed up a basket of nice things, and getting into the carriage, accompanied by Mr. and Mrs. Genella, we rode out to the lines, it was a long distance and though we had been

---

[84]An episode had taken place in Vicksburg between Father Heuze and several Black soldiers. They stormed into church on Pentecost, Sunday, 1864. Father preached at them; they stormed out of church and besieged the rectory demanding an apology. He would not; they withdrew, promising to get even. Three of them jumped him later but he survived.

[85]Major General Henry W. Slocum, New York.

[86]General Slocum exclaimed, "What, let Father Leray enter; I would as soon let in one of the Forrest's brigades." From unidentified newspaper clipping in Elder's file.

as short a time as possible, found that Father and his companions discouraged by their cool reception, had concluded we could not return, so
we were obliged to retrace our road, much to the dissatisfaction of the
black driver of the ambulance, who had begun to despair about the boots
and hats with which he had been pleasing his imagination and which
afterwards Mr. Genella and Clement[87] gave him.

Sunday morning after claiming our baggage at the Court House, we
started with two well filled baskets in the carriage. We found Father at
Mrs. Doctor Cook's. He had suffered much from anxiety about us. Poor
Mrs. Cook[88] looked like a heartbroken woman and walked with a feeble
step, the house had been literally dismantled of almost everything,
and the fear of the enemy had been the cause of the death of one of her
daughters; indeed, many of the young people of the country had withered
and died from the — blast of war. She would touch none of the things
Mrs. Genella offered, turning from the city of her enemies. After a few
moments' conversation, the Provost Marshall said they ought to go. We
bade farewell to Father Leray and the party. On our return the people
and children came to see us, welcoming Reverend Mother, especially,
with warmest affection.

The next day, Bennett, a man who had brought in our baggage
free of cost, being about to return, we presented a petition to Genl. S.
who, being in an amiable mood, and discovering he had known of Rev.
Mother previously in Washington,[89] granted our request to send out
things to the Sisters. We afterwards petitioned for our House, but he
said it suited him particularly well, on account of its proximity to his
own quarters, but promised to think of it; on our next interview he told
us he could not give us ours, but offered us another one. We declined,
as we could not take possession of anyone's property, except that given
by the Congregation, so he closed the interview somewhat sternly, as
neither the law, nor himself recognized, he said, our claims to any more
rights than any other citizen. We then requested room in the house,
which was then occupied by a woman, but it met with the like result.
The prejudice of this officer was not surprising as his uncle was a protector of the imposter, "Maria Monk," whom she rewarded by stealing his
silver and being imprisoned afterwards.[90] Nearly three weeks had now
elapsed, and we then wrote to Washington by request of our Bishop,[91]

---

[87]Clement Guidici.

[88]Minerva Hines Cook. Ironically, Mistress of "Hardtimes Plantation" outside of Vicksburg. She and
her 7 children were Catholic. Major Jared Reese Cook, her husband, was received into the church Sept.
10, 1863 by a Federal Chaplain, Father J. C. Carrier S.S.C., St. Paul Archives. Tradition has it that in
later years, a slave confessed to the death of her infant daughter.

[89]Probably at the Washington Infirmary. Rev. Mother DeSales had been in charge there before coming
to Vicksburg.

[90]A popular scandal autobiography about a nun who escaped the convent and told of atrocities experienced there. Very popular among anti-Catholics and "Know-Nothings."

who was, himself, then banished from Natchez, on account of refusing to say public prayers for the government.[92] We wrote to Honorable Francis Kernan,[93] under cover to Father [John] Early, President of Georgetown College,[94] giving a statement of our difficulties and requesting the possession of the Convent. In the meantime weeks passed on, the Sisters employed their time principally in study.

Mr. and Mrs. Genella were very kind, and Mr. Genella went himself to Genl. Slocum, who finally promised to let us have the house, when he should be removed.

Our letter to Washington did not reach it until Congress adjourned, but Bishop Michael O'Connor,[95] formerly of Pittsburgh, now a Jesuit, hearing of our situation, went himself to Secretary [Edwin M.] Stanton and obtained an order for the property, and on the 15th of August "Feast of the Assumption" after three months waiting, a document was sent us resigning the property by Genl. Slocum. We had made on the 24th of July an unsuccessful demand to have the woman whom we had left in charge of the place removed, but were harshly treated by the Genl., though we succeeded in getting a pass for Reverend Mother out of the lines with clothing for the Sisters; he refused rent for occupation of our house, but again, offered another house, and was a little more pleasant in the next interview. Reverend Mother, having borrowed a horse and buggy, was driven to Jackson by J.K., one of our former boys.[96] Having broken down by the way, they were obliged to proceed slowly[97] and arrived at 3 o'clock in the morning in Jackson, and were obliged to stand in the street, until day had broken sufficiently to find Mrs. Lucy's house, where they stopped and telegraphed to the Sisters,[98] who however, did not receive it in time, and Reverend Mother having left a trunk for them

[91]If they could not get the property back, the Bishop gave Sister DeSales three alternatives to ponder: take another house in Vicksburg, return to Shelby Springs, take refuge with the nearest Sisters of Mercy in Helena, Ark.

[92]Bishop Elder was banished across the river to Vidalia, La. and kept under surveillance there by Brigadier General Mason Brayman.

[93]A Georgetown graduate, Catholic from New York, a Democrat probably known by Sister Ignatius' brothers.

[94]Sister Ignatius' two brothers were Jesuits at Georgetown. John Early, S.J., helps greatly later in Elder's problems with separation of church and state.

[95]Bishop Michael O'Connor had been the priest in Pennsylvania who encouraged Sister DeSales to wait to enter the Sisters of Mercy, and he went to Ireland and accompanied the first Sisters to Pittsburgh. His own sister was a Mercy Sister.

[96]John Kearney, 12 year-old-son of Martin Kearney, brother of Sister Margaret Mary (only a baby at the time, having been born in a cave during the bombardment). The "Expanded Journals" describe John as "the lad, proved of great assistance more than once, in ways that boys alone can contrive."

[97]In the dark, through swollen creeks, being examined by sentinels."

[98]At Shelby Springs to meet her in Meridian 60 miles away.

at Meridian, sixty miles further, set out to return, fearing a raid might destroy the roads, and Sister Vincent and Father Leray were obliged to return without having seen Rev. Mother, a sacrifice for both.

Rev. Mother then went ten miles from Jackson to get the consent of the lady[99] (in case we should need it) to the occupancy of her house, which Genl. Slocum offered us instead of our own house. She returned, the same day to Jackson, and the next started for Vicksburg; but an under officer not being satisfied with her pass, she was delayed on her journey, until John Kearney could return to Jackson for a new one; but was kindly treated at the house she stopped at, where they refused to be compensated. She again experienced Mrs. Messinger's kindness, and arrived on Sunday, after ten days of incessant travel, exhausted, and worn out by fatigue. At last, after so much anxiety, our gracious Virgin Mother gave us our house, on her beautiful Feast [Aug. 15]. All the out-buildings had been burned down, the fence destroyed, the house injured, and trees destroyed, partly by Federal occupation, and partly by the family who were left in charge of it, when the sisters had first gone to take charge of the hospitals. Only too grateful to find themselves within the hallowed walls of the convent once more, the sisters began the arduous task of cleaning it, and of restoring its conventual aspect. In this they were assisted by their faithful ally, John Kearney, and one or two more of their former pupils, zealous, like him, for the comfort of the sisters. Their help was very opportune, since wheelbarrows and shovels were needed, rather than dust-pans, and brushes, or, brooms.[100]

"As the sisters had no means at their disposal except what they had borrowed for immediate necessities, a collection was taken up for them, at which six hundred dollars, which helped us along somewhat in the great expense we had to undergo in putting the house in order."[101] The Bishop, who had been banished to Vidalia [Louisiana], opposite Natchez, and his church threatened to be confiscated, was recalled, on the 23rd of August; after awhile, Genl. B. [Brayman] who had commanded in Natchez, was superseded, and he, himself, by a singular arrangement of Providence, was banished to the same place, for military misdemeanors.[102] The Bishop, however, was not allowed a pass to visit

---

[99]She was very scrupulous as a religious woman to occupy a house that was not theirs. In desperation she went to the trouble to secure permission from the owner in case Slocum went back on his word.

[100]John Kearney helped clean; Martin, his father, raised money.

[101]From "Expanded Journal" probably written in the hand of Sister Angela Fedou with the advice of Sister Ignatius Sumner, c. 1888, is used here, the original manscript of Sister Ignatius having deteriorated.

[102]Brigadier General Mason Brayman of Illinois. Slocum was angry for the convent ordeal. Both he and Brayman retaliated when Sister Thomas, Coronet Charity, requested rations for the orphans in Natchez. Brayman refused, sent his refusal to Slocum, whom he knew would approve of his actions; Genl. Slocum wrote a sarcastic letter saying "let Natchez take care of its orphans." Sister Thomas immediately wrote to Major Genl. Edward Canby, Union Military Commander of the Western Theater, stationed in New Orleans. He severely reprimanded Slocum reiterating to him that the Union government and soldiers had always been benevolent to the orphans.

us until November, when application was made to Genl. Dana,[103] who otherwise rigid and oppressive to the citizens, seemed well disposed to us. Margaret Ferrens,[104] who had been with us for more than three years, made a retreat, and was received by Father Charles Heuze, the devoted little pastor who had taken Father Leray's place during the siege and difficulties of Vicksburg. The school was reopened Sep. 12th [1864]. We had about two-hundred children, and at Catechism on Sunday, we averaged two hundred.[105]

Father Heuze, to the great regret of the people, as also of ourselves, left on the 20th of February, for the Novitiate of the Oblates of Mary, at Lyons in France, having long cherished a desire for the religious life.[106] Our holy Bishop came again, the Jan. before, 1865, to give us a retreat,[107] and at the renewal of vows on the 1st day, Sister M. Philomena having been admitted, nearly five years before, made her solemn Profession.[108] The Bishop gave us many conferences, and seemed to delight in being with us. During the six weeks he was here...ten converts, and brought back...[page has deteriorated here, bridge provided by "Expanded Journal."]

During his stay in Vicksburg, the Bishop gave the sisters several conferences, which served, not a little, to comfort and sustain them in the difficulties to which they were exposed, on account of fewness of numbers, want of means, etc. One of these conferences in which the Bishop chose for his subject "Fear not, little flock, for my Father has appointed you a kingdom," was particularly consoling, on account of its appropriateness to their own situation. Their numbers in Vicksburg was then only four. Rev. Mother prepared the sisters' meals, while they were in school, and when this work was over, lent her aid in teaching, visiting the sick, etc. Father [Patrick] McCabe, ordained in Ireland seven months before, came to take his place, [Father Heuze]. Shortly after came as pastor, Father Charles Von Quickleberge[109] [Van Queckelberge], who

---

[103]Maj. General Napoleon Jackson Tecumseh Dana had been wounded at Antietam. He was Union commander in Vicksburg, replacing General Slocum in August 1864.

[104]Became Sister Antonia at reception; at her vows, she took the name Sister Mary Joseph.

[105]400 children in all; many of the 200 who attend catechism on Sunday were from the levee immigrants, others were Blacks and children from outlying rural areas who do not attend during the week.

[106]A Religious Order offers more stability. Men take vows, live together in community. He entered the Marist Fathers at Lyons, France. He served in Dublin and London and Sydney, Australia, from 1869 to 1883.

[107]End of year three-day retreat.

[108]Final vows — perpetual for life. Postulancy was from 3-6 months to a year, then reception of name and habit; followed by one year of novitiate, then final vows. Sister Philomena Farmer had come several months after the original group from Baltimore. Temporary vows came later in canon law.

[109]A young Belgian priest from Louvain who came Dec. 1863 was allowed to work almost exclusively with newly freed Blacks, many of whom contracted smallpox. He contracted it, went to Cathedral in Natchez to recuperate. Elder took his place; he recovered and died from Yellow Fever in 1878.

had been delayed by ill health, contracted in attending the sick soldiers. Reverend Mother, who feared that a raid would prevent her from seeing the Sisters, went out once more to meet them in Jackson and Father Leray, with Sister Vincent, who was much changed, and broken, from a hemorrhage, came to see her, bringing a little Creole from N. Orleans, Aminaide Poursine, who had entered at Shelby Springs three months before. Reverend Mother brought her back with her, and arrived March 25.[110]

In the meantime, on March 12, about a hundred persons in all, and about seventy children of both sexes, had made their First Holy Communion and been Confirmed, after a retreat given by the Bishop. They formed a beautiful procession: the boys with white and red rosettes with white pants and black jackets, and the girls with white dresses, wreaths and veils, walked in perfect order, accompanied by two officers of the Sodality with their white ribbons, who attended to lighting and extinguishing their candles, which were tastefully decorated. The fathers made a public preparation and thanksgiving, before and after Communion, and the same at High Mass for Confirmation; in the afternoon, headed by three little boys they went to Vespers.[111] William S. [Smarr] read the Act of Renewal of baptismal vows, which [was] printed and decorated. He was supported on each side by one of the other two boys. The participants concluded by taking refreshments, accompanied by the Bishop and Fathers. Two of the Holy Cross Sisters[112] took breakfast with us in the morning, and our neighbor, Mrs. Quinn, sent us our Breakfast. In February, Reverend Mother concluded on account of our contracted space, as well as the necessity we had for the room, that we would have either to give up the boys, or build a school room, and as there was no other religious school, she concluded, though our means were inadequate, to build a school house, consisting of two rooms, which was accordingly finished, costing, though inexpensively built, $1500 or $2000. Sodality and Catechism were held there on the 9th [February].

Aminaide Poursine, after the usual retreat, was received April 6th by Father Charles [Van Queckelberge] as Sr M. Xavier. On the 30th of May, 1865, Peace having been declared, in consequence of the surren-

---

[110]Aminaide's family had been exiled from New Orleans by General Benjamin Butler. They settled in a little village near Shelby Springs. Aminaide joined in helping the Sisters at the hospital. She had to wait until the Sisters got established back in Vicksburg for her reception. Later her younger sister, Amelie entered. Father Leray and Sister Vincent returned to Shelby Springs. (See biography)

[111]Sang the introduction to the psalms and refrains. Probably trained by Sister Ignatius who taught music.

[112]The Holy Cross Sisters were nurses on a Union hospital boat "Red Rover" which plied up and down the river. They came before the siege, nursed Union soldiers during the siege, and kept the hospital boat and wounded soldiers until after the war. Many men were sick and dying from the fever. Sherman tried digging a canal to divert the river at Vicksburg to make a frontal assault. It did not work but got many sick with fever and dysentery. Father Elia, a Mississippi priest, worked with the sick and was the Sisters' chaplain. He died Apr. 3, 1863, from dysentery.

der of the Confederate Armies, the Sisters with Father Leray left the hospital at Shelby Springs, and after a journey of two weeks by way of Mobile and N. Orleans, being detained some days in the latter place, arrived in Vicksburg, after three years absence.[113]

On May 11, seventeen young ladies of the Sodality of the B.V.M. [Blessed Virgin Mary] were invested with the badge and medal, in St. Paul's Church, by Father Charles Van Quickelberge, who explained the advantages of a Sodality to the Congregation. Emma F. read the Act of Consecration, and the Sodality sang a hymn before and afterwards. Benediction concluded the ceremonies. They were dressed in white, with wreath, and veils, and lighted candles. On the Feast of the Purification, six young ladies of the Sodality of B.V.M. were Professed by Father Leray, who also gave them a little instruction at St. Paul's, and on the 16th of February, a Sodality of the "Angels of the Holy Childhood," erected by permission of Father Piot, their Director in this country, read their Act of Consecration and received the picture of the "Holy Childhood" from Father Leray, their local Director, to the number of thirty little girls, all under twelve years, except two or three.

Ann Keller from N. Orleans entered in June, Margaret Harrington of Washington entered the 4th of April, aged 18 years.[114]

On the 23rd of June, 24 girls and 20 boys made their First Holy Communion. Miss Kate Houck, aged 17, one of our former pupils in Baltimore, arrived Aug. 1st, was received Dec. 28th[115] on Holy Innocents by Rt Rev. W. H. Elder, who afterwards gave the annual retreat, closing on Jan. 1st 1867.

On Ascension Day, May 30th 1867, twenty-three boys and twenty-four girls made their First Holy Communion, having made their retreat under Father Leray. In the interval several postulants had been received and some dismissed.[116]

In May 1867, we had a Fair and a series of Tableaux designed by Miss H.S.,[117] a young lady from Baltimore, to enable us to purchase a piece of property, as we could not have the various objects of our Order, situated as we were, in such a small space. We realized about $4,500 which was remarkably good, as the people were suffering much at that time from the overflow of the river, loss of crops, etc.[118] Mr. Genella gave

---

[113]The Sisters were wearing rabbit-skin shoes, contrived by Father Leray. Their habits were held together with white thread.

[114]Both were received Nov. 21 as Sister Magdalen and Sister Veronica, both lay sisters.

[115]Sister Aloysius.

[116]Judged not suited for Religious Community because of character, temperament or work ethic.

[117]Helen Summer — the author's sister from Baltimore, nursed at Gettysburg, later married Jeff Davis Bradford, nephew of Jefferson Davis.

[118]A very bad flood year, 1867.

us the use of his picture gallery for the purpose. Sister Veronica, lay Sister,[119] died rather suddenly of a rapid consumption; she was a good and edifying Novice.[120] A devoted friend of the Sisters, Mr. [J.J.] Fitzpatrick,[121] attended to the funeral preparations. She was carried on a bier by the St. Paul's Society[122] with all the other Sodalities wearing badges covered with crape, as also were their banners trimmed with crape.

Eliza Martin entered from St. Louis, Aug. 1st, Received as lay Sister April 25th as Sister M. Germain, Feast of the Annunciation.[123]

Jane Corbitt came with Bishop Elder, from Baltimore, Dec. 8th on his return from Europe, Feast of Immaculate Conception. Received on Feast of the Annunciation Apr 23rd [sic] as Sister M. Catherine, Received earlier on account of her long tried virtues in the world, and her capacity for religious instruction, for which she was needed.

The Bishop gave us our three days' retreat ending Jan. 1st, 1868. The children welcomed him back, Will Smarr congratulating him in a speech, also a welcome song by the children. On the 18th of January Miss Bridget Murphy of N. Orleans entered, was received July 12th Feast of the Precious Blood, as Sister M. Angela.[124] She died suddenly Oct. 11th, at 25 min. to 10 P.M. of paralysis of the brain, caused by, we suppose, the disatisfaction and persecution of her family at her becoming a religious. Her edifying example was a great loss to the Novitiate.[125]

On the 17th of April, Miss Laura Stevens of Yazoo City entered, was received as Sister M. Rose Nov. 6th, 1868 and on the 19th of April Miss Teresa Kessel of N. Orleans, born in Germany, entered, received as Sister Gertrude at the same time as Sister M. Rose.

August retreat given by Father Meredith, C.S.S.R.[126] Rt. Rev. Wm. H. Elder returned from Rome after a year's absence. When he went away, Miss A. Katzenmier [sic], on the part of the school, and J.J. Fitz-

---

[119]Lay sister entered for domestic work rather than teaching.

[120]Sisters DeSales and Ignatius were in Chicago looking over buildings for ideas for the one to be erected in Vicksburg.

[121]A dear friend and benefactor of the sisters. He had moved from Meridian to Vicksburg and made arrangements for Sister's burial at St. Paul's church. He had helped the Sisters in Meridian.

[122]Men's fraternal organization similar to the Holy Name and St. Vincent dePaul, where the men joined in good works in the community, including being pall bearers.

[123]Feast of the Annunciation has been traditionally on Mar. 25 exactly 9 months to Dec. 25.

[124]Her parents had insisted on her marrying; she left home secretly and came to Vicksburg. Her parents learned of her whereabouts after she was received. Her mother came and tried to force her to return to New Orleans. Bridget refused but lived in dread of another such scene.

[125]She too was buried beside St. Paul's church. Sister DeSales was ill with pneumonia and unable to attend the funeral.

[126]Redemptorist priest.

patrick on the part of the Congregation, all present in the Convent yard, made the Bishop a speech, and presented him with purses amounting to over $700. On his return, Mannsell Mitchell,[127] made a speech of congratulation, and the children gave him over $100.

The cornerstone of the new Convent to be erected on our lot was laid Aug. 2nd, 1868, by Rev. F. X. Leray, under the patronage of St. Francis Xavier.[128] Two or three thousand persons assembled, to witness the Ceremony, and an immense procession was formed after Vespers, from the church, consisting of the Sodalities of the "Holy Infancy," "Angels of the Holy Childhood," "Blessed Virgin," "Altar Society," "St. Paul's Association," headed by the Post band, led by General [Alvan Cullum] Gillem. Father Leray made the opening address, followed by Mr. [William] McCardle, Editor of the "Times" and by Upton Young Esqr[129] — the music of the band, and the "Laudate Dominum," and "Magnificat" of the choir, filled up the interludes; it was Sunday evening, and as the moon rose slowly over the immense multitude, the whole scene formed a beautiful picture.

The Convent, planned by Father Mouton,[130] is in the Elizabethan style of Architecture, the assistance towards erection, Fairs, by kind assistance of Rev. F. X. Leray, P. Kennedy, and M. Kearney.[131] Building cost about $30,000. We took our first breakfast in the new Convent Christmas Day 1869. The first Mass said in our new chapel, Jan. 28th and 29th, the Feast of our beloved Rev. Mother. We were so crowded that the Sisters had to occupy some of the cells[132] before the Convent was finished. August 30th, 1869, 31 girls and boys made their First Holy Communion after a fervent retreat given them by Father Leray. 50 boys and 60 girls were Confirmed by Rt. Rev. Wm. H. Elder on Jan. 10th 1869 after Vespers on Sunday. Our Annual retreat was given by the Venerable Father Murphy S.J., ending on the Feast of the Assumption.

The one for the renovation of Vows ending Jan. 1st, 1869, was given by the Ver. Rev. Father Grignon[133] of Natchez.

[127]Nephew of Jefferson Davis.

[128]Named after Father Leray's namesake, Jesuit patron of the missions.

[129]Upton Young, a prominent lawyer, lived in the next block from St. Francis.

[130]John Baptiste, outstanding architect, also designed parish church in Columbus, Miss. presently standing.

[131]Martin Kearney, father of John Kearney, had a daughter. Josephine, born in a cave during the siege. She entered the Sisters in 1883 and became Mother Margaret Mary. Martin Kearney bought a piece of land adjoining the convent from an apostate who refused to sell it to the Sisters. It cost $4,500. Payments were made by fairs and cleared by 1878.

[132]Small sparse rooms occupied by Sisters.

[133]Mathurin Grignon came to diocese from France 1849 to be a professor at the seminary in Natchez. He was a learned priest. He was crippled. A well deserving clergyman, he was appointed Vicar-Genl. of the diocese in 1857. He served in Natchez.

Sister M. Aloysius Houck and Sister M. Magdalen Keller were Professed, Jan. 16th 1869 by Rt. Rev. W. H. Elder.

Misses Margaret and Emilia Hoey of N. Orleans entered May 13th 1869. They were both received Nov. 14th Margaret as Sister M. Alphonsus, Emilia as Sister M. Scholastica, the ceremony of reception was performed by Rev. F. X. Leray.

August Annual retreat had been given by Reverend M. Meredith, C.S.S.R., January retreat by Rev. F. X. Leray.

Mary Betz, Choir, and Augustine Essent, Lay Sister, entered Jan. 23 [1870], both from New Orleans. They were both received on the Feast of the Immaculate Conception, the first as Sister M. Benedict, the second as Sister M. Nolasco, by Ver. Rev. F. Leray, Reverend J.B. [Jean Baptist] Mouton preached on the occasion.

To revert to our Hospital at Mississippi Springs. The Sisters were invited to take charge of Mississippi Springs Hospital, which was at the time a fashionable watering place about forty miles from Vicksburg. No preparation had been made for us; we came right in upon the gay assembly, whose curiosity induced them to linger inconveniently long, until the Steward whispered something about Smallpox and then they took flight precipitately, leaving us such an accumulation of dirt to clean up, as we had never beheld. We had brought our own provisions and everything we had likely to be useful. It was well we did so. There were plenty of provisions at that time in the country; too little experience and forethought, besides some of the Officers were too busy making unto themselves friends of the Mammon of iniquity, to think of the needs of the sick, comforted only by what we could do for them, and give them, as many as 200, who were able to walk, escaped the general destitution by running off.

Our Medical head was a young man no doubt elegant in the ball-room and polished in Society, but quite out of place in a hospital; he gave directions every day for his dinner, our last chicken was sacrificed at his shrine. He understood not the wants of the suffering and reminded one of the gentlemen in another battle field who told the soldiers "they were most unmannerly to bring unhandsome corpses between the wind and his Nobility."[134] He forgot the friends now, who nursed him unweariedly for weeks.

His impractical turn is illustrated by a little anecdote ludicrous enough. The Steward was using his influence to get him to have a cover built over the soup boiler, which was in the open air, and he said: "Why

---

[134]Henry IV Part I Act I scene3 lines 40-45. Speech of Hotspur describing a popinjay acting in such a manner – Harry Percy.

Doctor, do you know I was walking towards the spot yesterday, and what should I see but two pigs smelling round and at last lift the pot off, shoulder it between them, and run grunting with pleasure away." "Is it possible, Tom?" says the Doctor. "Fact, Sir. I will have a cover by all means." The same man said to a sick soldier who wanted pants, "Not an article left, Sir. I applied to the Commissary the other day for a coat, and what did they give me, but a lady's ruffled skirt." The sick man looked at him aghast at this destitution, but said nothing. Our labors were very great. We had to go over long galleries and through a long ward to get a drop of warm water and the kitchen was literally a pig-sty. After some time we had a kitchen in our own portion of the building, and there Rev. Mother incessantly contrived little dishes for the sick. Father Leray was here with us. We had Mass and all our spiritual duties, except the Office. Many died of pneumonia and erysipelas. The first one who died was a Presbyterian. Sister asked him if he was satisfied with his religious belief; he said he had always wished to know and believe the truth; she showed him the Crucifix and explained what it symbolized, without disturbing him further as his time was short. No Catholic could have been more fervent in aspirations to his Crucified Redeemer, and his intuitive faith proved the circumstances of invincible ignorance and the charity of the Church which includes within her pale all who believe undoubtingly.

The next was a young Creole, who received the last Sacraments with pious dispositions, but felt deeply parting with his beloved brother, who hung over him in agonizing tenderness and whose grief, uttered in broken lamentations, made all around him weep. Sister said a Creole from the country perched on the foot of his bed like a monkey. "My Mother's cows have calved, and if I were home now I would give you some milk." The picture of rural pleasure was too much for him; he laid down and died the next day.

After some time our hospital surgeon was replaced by another, who was so rigid a disciplinarian that he preferred justice to mercy. Many were subjected to severe military punishments, and the convalescents were in such a state of starvation, that one night they tried to get him out to hang him. They were so little used to discipline; they felt it all the more repugnant to their ideas. In the meantime, many persons from the country round visited the hospital; at first from curiosity, or prejudice, but after some time, with better feeling, often bringing food to the patients, though it must be acknowledged, generally selecting the handsome fellows for the distribution of favors, so much so that the nurses [male] sometimes jumped in bed with boots on, so that some sentimental lady would bestow upon them preserves, and the gentle motion of the fan. One poor fellow, too sick and repulsive to attract a dainty notice, received the tenderest care of the Sister in charge; his next neighbor, who was not ill enough to require so much attention, complained to some bigoted woman; that he was not treated well, and she went to the Sister, taking her by the arm and shaking her. "Woman," said she, "How dare you treat a sick man so?" Sister made no reply, but the ill man, whispering in his dying voice, said, "Never mind, Sister, you do the best you can for all;" he felt the injustice of the accusation, though too weak to defend her.[135] A Sister was bringing some chicken soup to a poor fellow, the yellow victim of liver complaint. "Sister," said he, "Put that down a moment, and come here, I want something better." "What can you have better?" she answered. "Salvation," he replied. "There must be something in the religion which produces so much kindess." He wanted to believe the truth and said he had always prayed for it, and plain as he was in all exterior things, his soul was filled with trusting faith and upright simplicity. He was baptized next morning. How happy and full of peace he was! He was trying to sing at 6 o'clock in the evening and at seven he died.

[At this point, eleven pages are missing from the manuscript. The material continues as follows, during the 1878 yellow fever.]

Sister M. Agnes would have gotten well sooner but exerted herself before she was able, had a relapse and her illness was of five weeks duration, imminently in danger of death. In the meanwhile Sisters M. Angela, Josephine, M. Agnes Mills, Germaine and a postulant, afterwards Sister M. Baptista, were all ill and Sister M. Ignatius with a slight attack, also three girls in the house. The City Hospital physician [Doctor David Booth] feeling that he was becoming ill, offered the hospital to the Sisters; they took it under the direction of the "Howard Association,"[136] and they had about 300 sick. Most of those who were not brought there too late recovered, and many a soul who would otherwise have died without the Sacraments were prepared and fortified in that last struggle.

---

[135]In one of the hospitals a naive steward, convinced that the Sisters had been entrapped and were living in ignorance of the dangers to which their souls were exposed, kindly lent one of the nuns a copy of The Scarlet Lady, a book describing the horrors of convent life. To offset the good impression the Sisters were making on the soldiers they were nursing, copies of Maria Monk's Awful Disclosures of the Hotel Dieu Nunnery of Montreal 1st ed. N.Y. 1836, a vile attack upon the life of the Sisters in Catholic Convents, were circulated through the hospitals. Their service and actions spoke louder than printed word.

[136]Quasi-governmental agency, New Orleans Howard Association from 1837 to 1878 collected donations from New Orleans and the nation at large and dispensed aid to the sick and poor in the Crescent City and other towns in the region for 11 epidemics. They hired and assigned doctors and nurses in needy areas. Called Early Red Cross.

During all this time the Sisters who were able visited the sick from morning to night; many received the Sacraments and were baptized. Beef tea, chicken soup and jelly were constantly dispensed to the sick irrespective of creed while the Sisters almost forgot the requirements of nature themselves. The Sisters of Charity assisted us also in the hospital. Sisters with exception of two, took the yellow fellow and were brought home. Sisters M. Teresa and Scholastica were in Jackson afterwards joined by two others as soon as they were able to do so. The fever was not as virulent here[137] as in Vicksburg, but still, there was a great deal.

A School Master, who had a wife and children, lay dying in utter want and misery. "Father," he said to the priest who visited him, "I have waited for a message from the Master for five years, and this is what he has sent me. My family starving and in rags and I about to leave them. I want nothing to do with him."

The priest said not a word, but sent to the Sisters, and when he next came, the wife and children were decently clad; there was food and the house was clean and in order and the grateful and dying man lay clasping a Crucifix. "Now indeed, Father, I know how good God is and that he has not forsaken me." The poor fellow died in sentiments of compunction and resignation, having the promise that his family would be cared for. Donations had been showered upon the Bishop from the Bishops and friends from the North, which enabled him to help this family [be] clothed, and they were sent back to Massachusetts, their native State.

During the nearly six months our school was closed, we should have been unable to subsist ourselves but for the Bishop's assistance, aided by donations collected by the relations of some of the Sisters.

Sister M. Vincent at the close of our retreat had been sent to Meridian with three other Sisters and the parting was sad indeed, for there was a conviction on both sides that some of us would never meet again in this world. Meridian was quarantined, so they had to stay with Mr. [John] Semmes' family, ten miles in the country, for some time, where they were most hospitably entertained. They did not open school 'till Jan. 1st, though they returned to Meridian before that. Their culinary arrangements were of the most economical description. Bishop Leray[138] passed through to assist Vicksburg and they managed some batter cakes from their last flour, and sent them up to him with the last morsel of butter, about the size of a walnut; Sister Vincent, shocked at such a show of inhospitable meanness, immediately required the appearance

---

[137]According to the Jackson Sisters. The fever came often in Mississippi. In 1853 two promising young priests died attending the victims in Vicksburg: Father John Baptist Babonneau and John Fierabras, both recently ordained missionaries from France.

[138]Father Leray Apr. 22, 1877, consecrated Bishop of Natchitoches in 1879, named co-adjutor of New Orleans but administrator of Natchitoches until 1883 when he became ordinary of New Orleans. (see biography)

of more butter. The economical maker of cakes clasped her hands with a Melodramatic expression of despair and mildly, but mutely, appealed to Heaven. Fortunately for the discovery of her resources, the Bishop was too sick to eat anything. On another occasion, a Sister who knew nothing about being left to bake bread, she put a little statue of the Blessed Virgin in the back of the stove and her faith was rewarded by success.

Bishop Leray was exceedingly touched and overcome by the afflictions of the flock once his own. He also chartered a boat, took provisions and went to the Assistance of the Greenville Pastor who was ill. There were but fifteen survivors left in Greenville of those who had remained there. Meanwhile the Bishop and the Howard Association enabled us to assist many persons in Vicksburg. The deaths were variously estimated from 1300 to 1500, but we believe them nearer 2000, as many were buried at a time, and many in the country not in the Sexton's report.[139] We collected about 20 orphans and kept them until the juveniles were adopted by those who have proven devoted parents to them or put in suitable situations.[140]

The assistant priests, Father Oberfield and Father Huber,[141] were next down with the fever; six priests were already dead and about twenty Religious of various Orders in the Diocese. Six Nazareth Sisters of Charity had died in Holly Springs, one of them offering her life for the Bishop's preservation, two also were dead at Yazoo City and the rest ill when two of her Sisters, one of them just recovered from the fever, went up to nurse them.[142] They succeeded in saving the lives of the rest, except the Superior, Sister M. Lawrence, who was beginning to convalesce, when Rev. J. B. Mouton, their Pastor who had been a most zealous and self-sacrificing laborer amidst all the deprivations of an extensive country Mission, was taken with the fever, and died in a short time, his constitution having been already exhausted. Sister M. Lawrence seemed to receive a shock by the news, and died a few days after.

Two Daughters of Charity (Coronet) joined them there and returned with them when the balance of the Sisters had entirely recovered; they had but one bed between them, which each took in turn for some hours repose, as long as it was necessary to relieve each other with the sick and they made themselves very merry over the universal benefit one bedstead bestowed, being as one of them said, "Three religious orders,

---

[139]Population of Vicksburg 4,000. Funeral records show Sisters bought shrouds for many of the dead.

[140]Immigrants on levees had lost many fathers during the war. They were hard hit – "not an Italian to be seen" from Sister DeSales letters.

[141]Philip Huber, chaplain during war at major battles, had been pastor in Jackson. Father Herman Oberfeld had been pastor in Sulphur Springs from 1875. He became pastor in Vicksburg from 1879 to 1881.

[142]Sisters of Charity of Nazareth, Sisters of Mercy and Daughters of Vincent dePaul (Coronet Charities) all worked together to help each other here.

and but one community and one heart." Our school was opened in the middle of November. The fever had been particularly destructive to little children, as in almost every case it was combined with meningitis; and when the Sisters who had the infant school room went in that morning and missed thirty little familiar faces, she could not conceal her emotion, but wept over the lost, but now happy little cherubs. Nothing could have been a sadder or more striking contrast during the fever than the cloudless blue of the heavens; the softness of the air and the beauty of the nights, the moon looking down like the Angel of Justice, so lustrous, yet so coldly, upon the City of the dead. Houses closed, stores vacated, and often, except ourselves and the Physicians, scarcely a creature was to be seen, the inhabitants consisting of two classes, nurses and sick. On the whole extent of the levee on one day we saw one man sitting at the door; it had been always a swarming place, but the fever had been particularly fatal to Italians, most of whom lived here.[143] The convalescent Bishop Elder had been received with much joy at Natchez, whose people had offered incessant prayers for his recovery.[144] He had been appointed Coadjutor to the Archbishop of San Francisco, but he was afterwards, at the instance of the principal Bishops of the U.S., appointed to the Coadjutorship of Cincinnati, Archbishop Purcell being very old and feeble, and an active Bishop being necessary for the wants of that Diocese. The appointment was the greatest cross of his life. The Natchez diocese had been endeared to him by its poverty, his sacrifices, and the spread of religion, of which he had witnessed and been the instrument. Like those who part never to meet again, every little office of kindness towards us, protection of our interests, care for our welfare was thought of and performed. He left in May, being a most painful parting for both himself and the Community. One of our beloved Sisters, a great and holy sufferer who died four months after on Sep. 29th, was then sick, bade him good-bye and he said to her, "The Sacred Heart sends you this suffering," and she said, "Yes, pray for me, but you, you also are called on to suffer much in this trial." He had requested to have some Sisters sent to Canton, and though it was attended with great difficulties, and sacrifices, Rev. Mother sent Sister M. Agnes and three Sisters in the following September. The first house was found to be in inconvenient distance from the church, and the Pastor Father [Louis] Dutto[145], built a small room on the premises for boys. There were about 23 of the latter, the balance, girls, averaging 60.

---

[143]Levee in Vicksburg

[144]Cardinal Gibbons had erroneously received word of the death of the bishop, and prayers and masses for the repose of his soul had been offered.

[145]An Italian priest of rare energy, vision and charity. He wrote history and sociology, founded a neighborhood later in south central Jackson, bought land and subdivided it into lots for homes and gardens. The area is still referred to as Duttoville. He also established a brick factory.

After the epidemic was over, the City took back the hospital and requested the Sisters still to preside in Vicksburg and the hospital began to assume a more attractive appearance, the grounds being beautiful and cared for, and order, cleanliness and comfort of the sick being attended to with scrupulous care, so that, so far the hospital Committee, the Mayor and other officers connected with it have declared themselves satisfied.

The whole Vicksburg community with its various branches consists of about 40 Sisters, including Novices and lay sisters. Graduates are sixteen, including those of this year. Pupils for Music, Painting, and the languages keep their teachers constantly occupied. There is constant visitation of the sick, and instruction of adults, white and colored, are frequent. The Sodalities of the Blessed Virgin and Holy Angels each contain about 40 members. That of the "Infant Jesus" numbers about 150, eighty of whom are large enough to attend the meetings. There are occasional receptions in our chapel where infants receive their blessed badges from the hands of the pastor and in cases of funerals, processions of the Infant Jesus Sodality proceed from the church, with their banners, accompanied by marshals from the other sodalities, and accompany the funeral cortege some distance. The local houses have similar sodalities.

Several vocations have proceeded from the Sodality of the B.V.M. which consists of young ladies. The yearly First Holy Communion classes average about sixty boys and girls. They make a retreat of three days at the Convent and spend the whole of their First Communion day there.

Within the last two years the Brothers of the Sacred Heart have opened a College in Vicksburg on church property, which was commenced by Father John McManus and finished by Father Herman Oberfeld, which has removed the boys from our care.[146]

The jail in Vicksburg, and the Penitentiary in Jackson are frequently visited by our Sisters, and, while they often supply the savory Knic Knack or substantial morsel, instructions are given and books lent. Several conversions have been made, followed by baptism. Two of the most remarkable were that of a colored man at the close of the war implicated in the murder of his mistress in connection with a band of black soldiers headed by a white officer.[147] He was formerly carriage driver to his mistress and liked Reverend Mother, who often gave him something to eat, and one time saved him from punishment when he had stolen a pair of the Sisters' shoes.

---

[146]1880.

[147]Mrs. Reese Cook. Minerva Hines Cook, wife and mother of the Cook family who had given the Sisters hospitality on several occasions. She was brutally murdered by the drunken group of soldiers. She hid her youngest child under her hoop skirt when she was bludgeoned. She lived to the next day. Her husband was shot in the leg and ran to the adjoining plantations. Nine men were identified and hanged by military court for the murder.

She visited and instructed him when put in jail with eight others, and he seemed contented and recollected while the others were agitated. He was baptized and made his confession, and as he passed by the Convent standing on his coffin, Reverend Mother went out on the little front gallery and held up to him a crucifix, seeing which, he bowed his head, in token of resignation and crossed his arms on his breast. He was the only one who died composedly, saying a few words to the effect that he hoped his sins were washed away by the precious blood of his Savior.[148] The other case was that [of a] man who in a state of intoxication [had] murdered another. He had run away from his Mother at the age of eight years, born of ignorance and neglect. Religion alone could have given such dignity; faith alone such composure. Many were struck by it, and a few, we understood, converted.

In May, 1881, Bishop Francis Jansen, born in Holland and for years devoted parish priest in Richmond, was consecrated in Richmond, Va., by Archbishop Gibbons, Bishop Elder preaching on the occasion. He came immediately to his Natchez diocese. His kindness, frankness and simplicity of manner attracted all hearts and was a happy augury for the firm, kind, quiet and orderly administration which followed. He was received with an address of welcome by our children, accompanied by songs and Music. The same also in Jackson, where he shortly afterwards administered First Holy Communion and Confirmation. A feast was spread for himself, clergyman and children in the school house attached to the Convent, and he especially enjoyed the performance of the children for his benefit.

The pastor of one of the Missions had induced the former Bishop to consent to the Sisters being examined by the board of the public school at the request of the people that the school might get its quota of public money, and they be relieved from paying. The plan, as may be supposed, was extremely repugnant and embarrassing to the Sisters and contrary to the instruction on that head given in our "Customs."[149] Bishop Jansen at once relieved the Sisters from this shadow of a "bete noir," and forbade that the Sisters should be troubled by a similar proposition.

We should notice that our schools, though nominally pay schools, contain a large proportion of free scholars, no one being refused on account of inadequate means. That in Vicksburg averages nearly half, but on account of the close connection between families differently circumstanced, but of the same blood, we have found that one separate school could not be established without destroying the harmony of society, as our special Mission is amongst Catholic children.[150]

---

[148]He was one of nine hanged publicly in O'Neals Bottom presently (Harrison & 1st North St.).

[149]Customs of Sisters of Mercy. A book of directions governing ministries receiving and dispensing funds, spiritual activities, daily schedules, etc.

[150]Only the convent treasurer and principal knew who paid. Sisters of Mercy traditionally had pay school academies and free schools. St Francis was a combination.

The fiftieth anniversary of our venerated Foundress' profession, the Golden Jubilee of the Order, was celebrated Dec. 12, 1881. The Sisters of Mercy everywhere observed it as a solemn festival on which occasion High Mass was celebrated, sermons preached, special acts of Mercy performed, and in several places charitable institutions founded in order to celebrate more worthily and perpetuate the remembrance of the virtues of Mother McAuley. In Vicksburg a procession of the various societies came up to the Convent at 9 o'clock and accompanied the Sisters to the church, where High Mass was celebrated and a sermon preached by Reverend Father Picherit[151], who took his text from Judges, 5th chapter, "The valiant men ceased, and rested in Israel; until Debbora arose, a Mother arose in Israel." "There was not a shield on Israel and the spear lay broken on the ground." He compared Mother McAuley with this Mother in Israel, as she founded her institute at a time when Ireland was still suffering persecution for her faith, when religion grew silently in the shadow, under the hedges, and out of sight; dwelt upon her character, her sacrifices, her sufferings, and the immense amount of good she accomplished unostentatiously, her holy and patient life and holy death, the rapidity with which her Order had spread over the whole world, although she had no idea she was founding a religious Order; the lives of labour and deeds of Mercy which distinguished the members of her Order, and concluded by a graceful tribute to the Sisters in their midst, and as their presence forbade him to offend their modesty by further eulogy, he finished by a graceful. "I do homage to their deeds, and salute their virtues." After Mass, the procession returned to the Convent, and were invited to an entertainment in the evening, consisting of a play, comic speeches, a saluation to the "Catholic Knights" and some fine Music by the Sisters' pupils.

The Catholic Knights and Temperance Society then presented the Sisters by the hands of Doctor R. O'Leary in a short address, a beautiful silver chalice, gold plated, costing $200. The Ladies of the Altar Society presented, by Mrs. Doctor Mitchell,[152] who spoke beautifully on the oc-

---

[151]Father Henry Picherit was considered the great Confederate Chaplain. He brought medicines from New Orleans to the areas in need. He was arrested by the Federals for bringing caps for the ammunition. He claimed his French citizenship to be released (From M. J. Mulvihill. City Historian and father of Sister Claudia Mulvihill 1920.) He was the pastor who invited the Sisters to Jackson in 1870.

[152]Lucinda Bradford, niece of Jefferson Davis, second wife of Dr. Charles Mitchell. Her mother was Amanda Davis Bradford, sister of Jeff Davis; her husband was Catholic and she had converted to the faith and her children were Catholic.

casion, a fine, life size statue of Our Lady of Lourdes, in the attitude she took in replying to Bernadette's question of who she was, "I am the Immaculate Conception,"[153] was having a rosary of white stones on her arm. It cost $80. They were then all invited to the parlors, where long tables of various refreshments were spread; and the day became doubly memorable to the Sisters of Mercy.[154]

Dear Rev. Mother, Please keep these manuscripts for us after you have finished with them as all the latter part is from memory and we have no other Record than this, which may be interesting to our Sisters at some future time, if preserved.

> Affectionately yours,
> Sister M. Ignatius,
> Convent of Mercy,
> Vicksburg.
> April, 1882.

---

[153]The Lourdes devotion was in popular vogue at the time.

[154]On her death bed, in Baggot St. (Ireland), Catherine McAuley ever sensitive to the care the fatigued Sisters were giving her, admonished them "to be sure that all the Sisters are given a comfortable cup of tea when I am gone," thus Mercy Sisters provide refreshments and hospitality.

Sister Mary DeSales Browne
1826-1910

The miracle of Catherine McAuley's Sisters seemed to be in the increase and spread of the order throughout the English speaking world. The Browne family of Pennsylvania certainly made their American contribution of four daughters: Fannie, Teresa, Mary, and Martha to become Sisters DeSales, Regina, Joseph, and Vincent respectively.

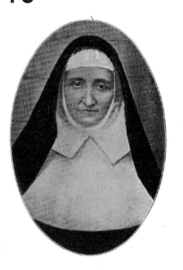

Westmoreland County, Pennsylvania's hills were the home of Michael and Mary Browne who were financially stable and lived like "the early Christians in piety and simplicity."[1] They had four girls and a boy and had to travel many miles to Mass. Missionary priests soon learned of this family and the hospitality of Mother Browne as she was lovingly called. Bishop Kenrick called her the "Apostle of Western Pennsylvania."[2] She instructed neighborhood children and prepared them for the sacraments. Her oldest daughter wanted to become a Religious Sister. Her pastor, Father Michael O'Conner, encouraged her to wait until the Sisters of Mercy came from Ireland. In 1843 Father O'Conner went to Ireland to accompany Sister Francis Xavier Warde and the first group of Sisters of Mercy to America for a Pittsburgh foundation. Fannie, at age nineteen, was one of the first postulants. Her three sisters followed her example, one by one. Sister Mary Vincent was her companion on the Southern mission. Sister Regina died during the height of the Civil War serving in the Washington Infirmary. Sister Mary Joseph entered the Buffalo, New York, community as the first postulant in 1861 and served there in leadership positions until her death in 1917.[3]

Fannie learned the Mercy way from those Irish Sisters near and dear to Catherine McAuley, the foundress of the Sisters of Mercy. A hardy American with both American and Irish roots both spiritual and temporal, Fannie Browne thoroughly imbibed the true Mercy spirit of service to the poor, sick, and uneducated. In total abandonment to

God, Fannie Browne, now Sister DeSales, set out in 1860 on her Mercy Apostolate with a fervor that led her on a path which would span the works of Mercy and the South.

Sister DeSales was a most attractive person, spiritually and physically. When the motherhouse in Ireland requested a picture of a representative native American Sister a photograph of Sister DeSales was sent.[4] She began her Mercy ministry at the Orphan Asylum in Pittsburgh and continued to fill posts of responsibility in Pittsburgh. She received thorough training in Mercy Hospital, Pittsburgh, where she studied under two Doctors McGirr, the father and brother of Mother Vincent McGirr and became a well-trained surgical nurse.[5] In 1852 Sister DeSales had been sent there along with four other Sisters (Sisters Isidore Fisher in charge, Angela McGreary, Stephana Warde and Colette O'Conner). Next the Pittsburgh Sisters took over the Washington Infirmary (located between Fourth and Fifth Streets, F to G in District of Columbia). This was also a teaching hospital with a faculty of distinguished physicians of the day. In 1855 Sisters Isidore and DeSales returned to Pittsburgh for elections. Sister DeSales returned elected as administrator of the Infirmary, accompanied by her sister, Mary, now Sister Regina. Also in 1855 three Sisters led by Sister Catherine Wynne came to open a school. In 1856 Sister Camillus Byrne, Mother Catherine McAuley's godchild, was sent to help. Because of the distance between Pittsburgh and Baltimore, in 1858 Baltimore was made a separate foundation with nine professed Sisters and seven postulants. The seven postulants in 1855 and 1856 were Sisters Joseph Medcalfe, Alphonsus Atkinson, Lucy Duffy, Stanislaus Matthews, Ignatius Sumner, Agnes Moran, and Vincent Browne.[6]

Sister DeSales suffered some health problems in 1859, and she convalesced at the school convent in Baltimore. While she was recuperating there, Bishop William Henry Elder of Mississippi applied for Sisters for a school for his most populous Catholic city, Vicksburg, Mississippi. Sister DeSales was chosen to lead a group of six Sisters in October of 1860 to start a school. The oldest of the group at thirty-four, she started on the pilgrimage of a lifetime. A naturally timid person, Sister DeSales, on being chosen for leadership, said in later years, "I tried to remain perfectly resigned to God's Will, in spite of the feeling that with my ill health I was unfit to establish our order so far away; but the thought that I would have to bear this cross only for a short time, since my frail body indicated a journey to heaven rather than to Mississippi, I calmly awaited until the burden of administration would be laid on abler shoulders."[7]

Her new pastor and co-worker was Father Francis Xavier Leray, a very assertive authoritarian priest; for years to come he and Sister DeSales seemed to complement each other. Her gentle compassion and desire to serve the neediest, while always thoughtful of her fellow sisters, melded well with his outspoken abrasive manner. He protected the Sisters but exacted much from them. As Sister Ignatius Sumner organized the school, Sister DeSales immediately discovered the wretched homes of the new immigrants on the "levee," one of her favorite spots for visitation. After a successful two years in school and the entrance of a fine Vicksburg lady, Sister Teresa Newman, war exploded between North and South. Gunboats began bombarding the River City. The Sisters were afraid. Sister DeSales reassured them and chose to accept the Confederate Army's invitation to nurse wounded soldiers. Bishop Elder insisted that a priest stay near the Sisters for their protection and spiritual service, so through Sister DeSales' efforts, Father Leray was permitted to accompany them. In consulting with Father Leray, he encouraged her to leave the novices free to return to their homes. He also said, "You have given yourself to God, and He is bound to take care of you." These words invigorated and comforted her during her new task. Another encouragement was the noble offer of Sister Ignatius to remain instead of returning to Baltimore since she was only lent to the new foundation.[8] Sister DeSales' attitude was always to serve where the need was greatest.

The care of those in need was the first order of business of the Sisters. In Washington Sister DeSales comforted and helped a prostitute dying of syphilis to die in peace; in Oxford, Mississippi, she chopped wood in the night to provide fire and warmth for wounded soldiers from the Battle of Shiloh. She set the example of service, compassion, and Christian love. The Sisters' example was a constant confrontation to those exploiters gaining from the war. She was courageous in making decisions to separate the Sisters. When the Bishop insisted she and the other Sisters come back to Vicksburg in 1863 to reclaim their property occupied by the Federals, she left half of the Sisters in Shelby Springs, Alabama, where they were needed to nurse the wounded. She followed her heart but could rationalize that she was following the Bishop's early directions to her, "Don't go out all together; I do not want you all to be killed. Divide and work in different directions so that some of you may escape."[9] How she must have hurt when she received the letter at Shelby Springs that her dear sister, Sister Regina, had died October 30 nursing in Washington.

Her meetings with General Henry Slocum in which she confronted him in her forlorn attire and rabbit-skin shoes, must have presented a picture of contrast to his arrogance and rudeness. Her tenacity in going to the top for justice, and her persistence in not using another's property without their permission showed her sterling character. What a sight! She and twelve-year-old John Kearney traveling from Vicksburg to Jackson and back, being stopped and interrogated by Union sentinels in their efforts to secure an alternate dwelling place for the Sisters in the event Slocum would not return the convent. How she must have spent a night in dread worrying when John had to return alone to get the proper passes. Another dread was that the Sisters should be compelled to go shoeless and in calico dresses (cheap cotton fabric with figured patterns) since one of the postulants, Sister Margaret Ferrens, was in dire need of a dress which cost several hundred dollars in Confederate money.

When she finally got the property evacuated of Federal troops, the school was reopened in 1864 with 200 students and only four Sisters, Ignatius, Philomena, Margaret Ferrens. Father McCabe helped teach; it was Sister DeSales who prepared the Sisters' meals, taught, and visited the sick. She left the other Sisters where they were needed in Shelby Springs. Sister Mary Vincent, Teresa, Agnes, Stephana and Xavier Poursine remained nursing.

After the war she served as superior and directress of novices. Many young women entered. She was a perceptive judge of fitness for religious life. She could often be found helping in the kitchen and laundry. The bishop sent many young priests whose health was threatened, to Vicksburg, because he knew her healing powers. She would treat them with strengthening tonics and appetizing foods. She was an avid reader and would remail Christian magazines and papers to families in the rural areas. She took in two retarded girls, one from a wealthy Bolton family; one penniless from Natchitoches, Louisiana.[10]

Her wide arms and loving heart included all. In Reconstruction times, a Black carriage driver was accomplice to the murder of a dear friend and benefactor of the Sisters. Sister DeSales faithfully visited him in the city jail, no doubt an unpopular gesture with the population. She prepared him for death and enabled him to journey to the gallows reconciled to God and with dignity.[11]

His wagon passed by the convent where she was standing with her crucifix held up for him to view. Nine United States Colored Troops were courtmartialed and hanged in O'Neal's Bottom, two blocks from the convent. All passed the convent, bound and standing in wagons.[12]

In 1869, Sister DeSales showed her traditional hospitality when she and Sister Ignatius in the carriage of their friend Captain J.J. Fitzpatrick went to the waterfront on Good Friday, March 26 to greet the "Mollie Able" steamship. Aboard were the six Sisters from St. Louis who were on their way to New Orleans to start the Mercy foundation there.[13]

Leader of the group was young Sister Catherine Grant; one member was Sister Austin Carroll, the Mercy author. They stopped for a visit at St. Paul's Church on the way to the convent. They visited with the Sisters at St. Francis for several hours. Sister Austin Carroll recorded in her annals that Sister DeSales gave them souvenirs, books, catechisms, medals, and rosary beads. She also presented gifts to the captain of the boat and his family.[14]

Almost exactly three years later, young Sister Catherine Grant reappeared in Vicksburg in the last stages of tuberculosis and asked Sister DeSales to give her hospitality once more. Characteristically Sister welcomed her again, and after three weeks, the recipient of the kind ministrations of the Vicksburg Sisters, breathed her last and was the first Sister buried in the convent cemetery.[15]

Her indefatigable leadership at the public hospital during the yellow fever epidemic was an example for all. Dr. David Booth, the administrator, made as his dying request a plea for the Sisters to take over City Hospital. Never to say no to a need, Sister DeSales wore herself out with work. At the hospital, the Sisters nursed as many as three hundred patients a day. Her letter to Sister Austin Carroll of New Orleans describes the height of the plague:

> *The fever here is of the worst character I have ever seen Deaths frequently occur in a few hours. Whole families have been swept away. There is scarcely an Italian left in the city. We found a dead body in every house on the levee. The City Hospital has been turned over to us, and our Sisters from our other houses have come here to aid us. The whole place is a desert. Not a human being to be seen in the streets, save the black-robed Sisters hurrying on their mission of mercy, or some member of the benevolent societies. From morning till night, good Bishop Elder is to be found at the bedside of the dying, administering the Sacraments, consoling and encouraging all. If he gives himself any rest these days, no one knows when. Pray God to come to our aid. He alone can help us now.[16]*

The Bishop was quarantined in Vicksburg. All the priests had died or were sick before the epidemic was over. Bishop Elder became sick, and his death was rumored. Cardinal Gibbons said a Requiem Mass for him. Sister DeSales too, became sick with the fever, but suffered most over the death of six of her dearest Sisters who served in the hospital. It was characteristic of Sister DeSales to be brief; she said much in a few words as indicated by this letter to her Sister in Meridian:

> *Vicksburg*
> *Convent of Mercy*
>
> *October 2, 1878*
>
> *Sister M. Vincent*
> *My dear Sister:*
> *Have pity on me, have pity on me, for the hand of the Lord*
> *hath touched me. I see my little community devastated by*
> *this dread pestilence. Let us trust God. Pray for them, pray*
> *for me. Our dear Father, Bishop Elder, is ever consoling*
> *and helpful. He reminds us of the saints of old as he walks*
> *through the streets and byways with the confessional stole*
> *on his arm, helping the priests to shrive and comfort the*
> *dying. May the little community in Meridian be spared if it*
> *be God's will. Your affectionate mother in Christ,*
> *Sister M. DeSales*[17]

This letter was written less than a month after Sister Bernadine Murray had died on September 7. The Brownes had one brother, Joseph; Sister Bernadine was his sister-in-law; she had entered from Dubuque, Iowa, December 21, 1877. She remained a postulant for five months, was received as Sister Bernadine on May 24; four months later she died of the fever. Four Sisters died that one week in September. What a poignant loss for the Browne sisters was the death of Sister Bernadine.

In serving the needs of those who most needed help, Sister DeSales was always ready to take risks. She showed undaunted faith in God and placed financial concerns in God's hands. Needless to say, she must have had some financial anxieties. Expansions were made in Vicksburg immediately after the war. Classrooms had to be built for the boys. Lumber had been stolen so, two thousand dollars had to be spent to replace it, even for the rough structure that was erected. In 1869 Pass Christian foundation was opened. The convent was paid for by the Sisters themselves; the land was purchased from the church. The pastor,

Henry Georget lent some money to the Sisters which was paid back without interest.

In 1870 the Sisters went to Jackson, and in the first two years paid one thousand dollars on the property for the school and convent. In 1872 for a nominal sum, Bishop Elder transferred the property to the Sisters on the condition that they teach poor children of Jackson; if they should cease teaching these children, the church could buy the property back for the original purchase. The school was closed for six months in 1871 because of the fever, and the Sisters had to depend on donations from relatives.[18]

With the expansion of two new foundations and the opportunity to buy adjoining property in Vicksburg, Sister borrowed $4,000 from Father Leray. Martin Kearney handled most of the transactions, and he donated $6,000. Father Leray did not ask for payment until he became bishop of New Orleans in 1876. Payments were made by money donated, earned from the school, and by fairs and plays. From 1876-1887 when Sister was sending small payments, she always wrote a personal letter. This one shows her humility:

Feb. 11, 1884

Most Rev. Bishop Leray:
Dear Father,
Enclosed please find check for four hundred. You will, I hope, pardon the delay; as you have doubtless heard of the failure of Klein's bank which has affected a great many of our people, some left penniless, a great many indirectly injured. Please dear Rt. Rev. Father for the sake of the holy relationship that has existed between you and our beloved community do not tell Mother Austin of any of our affairs. I am a poor ignoramus whom our dear Lord has chosen to make use of. Asking your prayers and blessings for me and mine.
        Devotedly in Christ,
        Sister DeSales[19]

This woman, who as a young Sister was ready to accept an early death, went on to celebrate her 50th anniversary in 1898 and lived 13 years after that. She outlived her five original companions and died at age 84.

The jubilee celebration was the happening of the year in Vicksburg, Mississippi. Bishop Elder, now Archbishop of Cincinnati, "one of the most

most learned and eloquent men in America," despite his advanced age of 79 years, came and gave the address.[20] Elder, 1819-1904, died at age 85, outliving Sister DeSales by a year. A religious statue was given on behalf of the city of Edwards for the services of the Sisters who nursed there during the yellow fever epidemic the previous year. A highlight of the event had to be the attendance of Indians from the newly established Choctaw mission. How proud Sister DeSales must have been to see the two Indian young ladies Minnie Jack and Louise Sucky present the elaborate spiritual bouquet and letter in Choctaw accompanied by the English translation. In their native colorful dress they joined the procession to the church. Surely the Sisters had prepared them as carefully as possible for this venture into jubilee celebrations, but the Choctaw girls had never seen steps and about 50 steps surrounded the entrance of St. Paul's Church which was constructed on one of Vicksburg's hills. They surprised everyone present and surely brought a smile to Sister DeSales face when they proceeded to mount the steps on all fours just as they climbed trees in Neshoba County.[21]

The year of her jubilee 1898 marked the establishment of seven schools and convents and the administration of the City Hospital. The number of the Sisters had grown from the original six to 56. By her death in 1910, 12 schools and convents had been established by this pioneer Sister of Mercy. Another hospial, the Gulf Ship Island Railroad Hospital, opened in Hattiesburg for injured employees and typhoid fever victims. Three Sisters supervised this hospital from 1902-1905.[22]

The sensitivity of Mother DeSales to a love without reserve can best be expressed by an excerpt from a tribute at the golden jubilee by John Brunini, the late Bishop Joseph Brunini's father and prominent Mississippi lawyer:

> *... Need I recite to you her work among us? No, let rather*
> *the countless homes tell you of the blessings they have*
> *received at her hands; look at the unalloyed expressions*
> *of gratitude that light up the countenances of her band of*
> *pupils, some of whom are now fathers and mothers and*
> *grand-fathers and grand-mothers; aye, let the poor of your*
> *city speak, visit your prisons, spend a minute at the hospi-*
> *tals, listen to the repentant sinner, go to the sick chamber,*

linger a moment at the deathbed, unfasten the lips of the victims of your deadly epidemics, and above all, let the little orphans with their tender and innocent little smiles whisper their praises, and you will appreciate the magnificient trophies that she has laid.[23]

Sister Mary Vincent Browne
c. 1836-1883

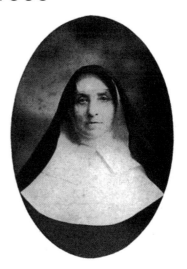

In the history of the Sisters of Mercy in Vicksburg, Sister Mary Vincent often remained in the shadow of her older sister, Sister DeSales. Possessing a keen sense of humor and a fund of common sense, Martha Browne, the youngest daughter of this pioneer family, began her initiation journeys for the Lord as an infant. She was carried sixty miles in a sleigh in Westmoreland County, Pennsylvania, to be baptized.[1] After the death of her mother, she entered the community following her three Sisters: Fannie (Sister Mary DeSales), Mary (Sister Mary Regina), Teresa (Sister Mary Joseph). She entered in Baltimore at the same time as Fannie Sumner and the five other young aspirants who became great leaders in Baltimore, under the tutelage of Mother Catherine Wynne and Sister Camillus Byrne. Her vows were made in a private ceremony, the Archbishop having advised against public ceremony because of the hostilities of the Know-Nothings, an anti-Catholic group who burned convents and schools. She was a young woman of robust health, and as a postulant, she was given the duty of visitation of the sick in their homes. The area of their parish was full of poor working people and soon became four parishes. Soon after Martha's profession, Catherine Wynne had surgery for cancer. It seems Sister Mary Vincent was her nurse, and she strained herself and undermined her health — so that she suffered a hemorrhage. She, along with her sister, was chosen for poor health reasons to go to the genial climate of the Southern Missions.[2]

Sister Mary Vincent was chosen to teach the boys, and she proved most talented for the charge. The perfect mixture of discipline and kindness seemed to be hers to deal with male students. And there was an initial announcement in the Vicksburg paper assuring parents that the boys would have an entirely separate school:

THE SISTERS OF MERCY
Have the pleasure to announce the opening of their
Academy for young ladies, and likewise of a school for
boys under twelve years of age.
Both departments will be perfectly separate and distinct
and care will be taken in each to ensure to parents and
guardians every advantage of a solid and polite education
to the children under their charge.[3]

One incident is told of Father Leray conducting the three-day strictly silent retreat preceding First Communion for the teenage boys. After the boys had made their first confessions, one mischievous fellow stood on his head in the middle of the room and caused the group to laugh. Sister Agnes Maddigan, not quite the disciplinarian that Sister Mary Vincent was, shuddered. Sister Mary Vincent returned, investigated the incident, and pardoned the offender discerning that no malice was intended, only an expression of joy in being unburdened of his sins. Sister Mary Vincent was considered fair and would give a fellow a second chance. She also taught boys at night and at Sunday school.[4]

The Kearney family was close to the Sisters, especially to Sister Vincent. John Kearney, a ten-year-old youngster, was one of the twelve children of this family who had come to Vicksburg from Baltimore as the first settlers. The family lived only a few blocks from the convent. On the Sisters arrival, John was chosen to welcome the Sisters with a large basket of pantry supplies. He had never seen a Sister. He left the basket at the door, knocked and ran to the outer walk. Sister Vincent opened the door and spent time convincing John that she was real. Here they became fast friends and John became a fathful ally of the Sister throughout his life. Sister Vincent taught him in the first class in school. He helped in the kitchen, brought berries, fruit for preserving by his goat team from the woods. John's dedicated love and service to Sister Vincent and the Sisters of Mercy indicated the influence Sister Vincent exerted in the community, especially with boys who went on to become leaders. John accompanied Sister DeSales to and from Jackson, during the war in attempts to reclaim the property. He smuggled the Sisters and priest through to Jackson during the 1878 yellow fever epidemic. He was at the time a member of the Howard Association, the group which aided the yellow fever victims. He was always listed in later years as pall bearer for deceased Sisters. Thus began Sister Vincent's ministry as teacher of boys.[5]

During the war, she was always designated "the superintendent of nurses" or the nurse in charge. A diplomat and a keen negotiator, she could mix seriousness and a sense of humor. Her care of the wounded men was compassionate and professional. Many a young man she consoled in death, and many a letter she wrote to widows and children informing them of their loved ones' last hours, death and burial. Years after the war, she received letters from soldiers she had nursed expressing their gratitude. In her humility and modesty, she would read a letter and share it with the Sisters and then destroy it.[6]

She experienced some bigotry too. On one occasion, a young man roughly mangled and dying was brought in. He had been a Catholic from birth, but war had made him angry and bitter. Sister Mary Vincent tried to console him, pray with him, and help him to die a peaceful death, but his last response was of anger and frustration. She felt grieved and disappointed. The man in the adjoining bed, who had been previously reticent and uncooperative, having witnessed this scene, called to Sister and asked her "to forgive his rudeness and teach him how to pray," which she did. Before many days, he went to God in peace with Sister at his side. This was probably one of many incidents.[7]

She was always left in charge when Sister DeSales left for any purpose. During the long separation when DeSales went to Vicksburg after the surrender in July, 1863, to reclaim the property, Sister Mary Vincent held the group together in Shelby Springs, Alabama. She practiced heroism during the long days of uncertainty. While doing double duty without the Sisters who had gone to Vicksburg, she cheered the young sisters and women volunteers, always making a joke of their many privations.

Sister Ignatius notes that Sister Mary Vincent was changed and broken again from a hemorrhage when she met Sister DeSales in Jackson in '63. After the war, she was the one to set up each new school and stay with the group until everything was going smoothly. In 1876 she went to Port Gibson to begin the mission; it failed, and she went in 1877 to Meridian after which she was to return to Jackson. In Meridian, the priest had purchased a discarded dry goods store for the convent. Four Sisters were met by a cabman who flippantly said, "This way to the poorhouse." She likewise retorted, "Take us to St. Aloysius Academy, I am the porter of that establishment," and he took them to the dilapidated building where it rained heavily, and the roof leaked all night. Her companions on this mission often recalled the many little circumstances in which her keen appreciation of the ridiculous turned a forlorn event into a subject of laughter.[8]

When the community in Vicksburg was ten years old, Sister Mary Vincent was sent to establish Pass Christian, the first branch house. It is interesting what the statistics then were: Entered 22, Dismissed 8, Dead 4, Total Members 20. This was 1870, a year of activity for Sister Mary Vincent. She and Sister Philomena Farmer and two companions went by boat down the river on the Steamboat *Natchez* to New Orleans then on to the Gulf City over Lake Pontchartrain on another boat to the Pass. This took a week. The highlight of the trip was their overnight stay "with the Sisters of Mercy on St. Andrew St., New Orleans, and the life-long friendship which was formed with the saintly Mother M. Austin Carroll," (author of the annals of the Sisters of Mercy)[9].

This beautiful seacoast mission had Corpus Christi processions. The Sisters taught, cared for the church, and made altar breads. The Sisters taught mostly children of fishermen and those who worked in the summer resort houses of the wealthy. Both Black and White schools were started with the enrollment about 60 boys and girls in each school. The school for Black children remained until the Josephite Fathers came. Nine months after the foundation, Sister Mary Vincent was recalled to lead the new mission in September in Jackson with five Sisters. In October 1871 one of the yellow fever epidemics broke out in the Federal Barracks at Jackson. Three of the Sisters attending the barracks were stricken as well as the pastor, Father H. Picheritt. Sister DeSales went to Jackson to nurse the Sisters and stayed until they grew better. Sister Mary Vincent was brought to Vicksburg, to recuperate. The school in Jackson was closed and not re-opened until January. Recurrent yellow fever episodes interrupted Sister M. Vincent's ministry in education.[10]

A statement in the annals says, "she neither feared pestilence at home or violence abroad."[11] She was there to bring peace and comfort to the parting soul. She was caught on several occasions in her travels because of the quarantine. Another terrible epidemic hit in 1878 when she was sent to lead a group to the convent in Meridian. Because of the fever, the Meridian town leaders established a "shot gun quarantine." The Sisters were unaware of this when they boarded the train in Vicksburg. Ten miles out, the conductor pitched their trunks off the train and said they had to get off. Sister M. Vincent said they had paid their way to Meridian. The conductor replied his orders were to let no one off at Meridian. In her astute manner, she looked at his timetable and list of stations and picked the station immediately before Meridian, a small town called Chunky. She told him, "We'll get off at Chunky; it has a comfortable sound." Her young Sister companions were nervous. She calmed their fears, but they were let off in a lonely spot in total darkness.

Luckily, the flagman had been one of her former students; he left a good lighted torch. True to her deep faith, she was rewarded with hospitality in Chunky until they could get to Meridian. There they were guests of the John Semmes family for 14 days.[12]

After many trips between Meridian and Jackson, Sister Mary Vincent was ready in 1880 to take on her fifth and last branch house. This time the place was Canton, the place where they had been in boxcars with 900 soldiers in 1863. The town now had wealthy families, aristocratic citizens, parents who were quite particular about the status of their children's teachers. From the beginning, the Sisters did not have the usual struggles with poverty. The first year was prosperous and pleasant; here was a large Catholic parish composed of well-educated parishioners. Surely Sister Mary Vincent was out of her element in this environment; she didn't stay long. The consumption had gained a strong hold on her. She would not let the Sisters write to Sister DeSales of her declining health. In her ever-optimistic way, she hoped later to rally as she so often had before. Finally, she had to be brought back to Vicksburg the latter part of 1882. The Sisters were startled at her appearance. She remained confined to the infirmary in great pain. The Sisters describe her during her last illness as a "valiant woman."[13] Her great motto had been "Never to ask, nor to refuse."[14] Her sunny temperament and ready wit lightened her last days. This time, however, she would not rally and arise with renewed vigor as she had done so many previous times.

She died in January of 1883 at age 47; this pioneer initiator. She was a perfect model of a Sister of Mercy going where most needed, her spirituality mixed with good humor. She was the low-key lady always moving on. Her remains were affectionately laid to rest by six of her former pupils, one of whom was her first student John Kearney.[15]

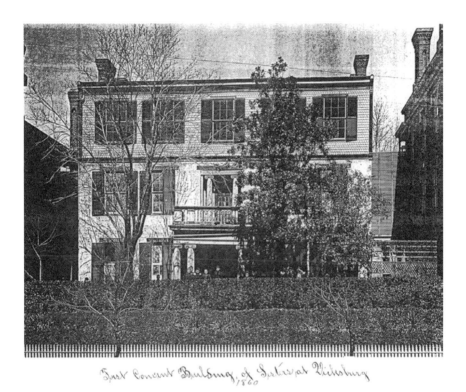

First Convent Building of Sisters at Vicksburg
1860

First building of the Sisters in Vicksburg, St. Catherine's, originally the Cobb Home on Crawford Street. The top story was removed later. Note the hedges to spare the view of the neighbors from the shanty-boat Irish children. This building was used for the convent, school, and temporary hospital.

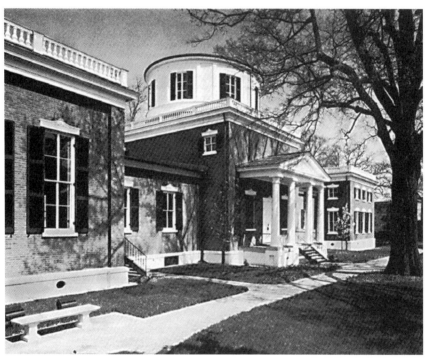

Courtesy <u>*The Southern Register*</u> *Newsletter of Southern Culture Center*
University of Mississippi

The Barnard Conservatory, used for a hospital by the Sisters, is presently restored and used for the Center of Southern Culture Studies at the University of Mississippi. Story has it that Grant knew Professor Barnard and so did not destroy the building.

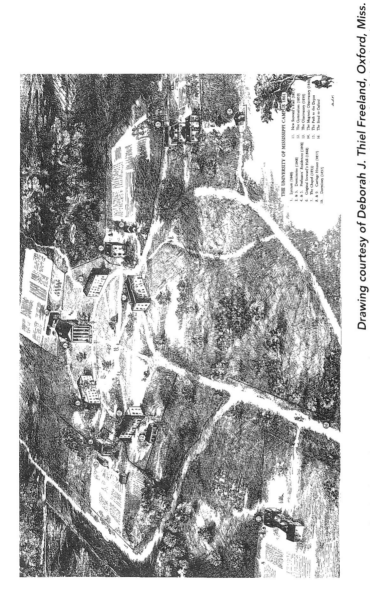

THE UNIVERSITY OF MISSISSIPPI CAMPUS 1861

1. Lyceum (1848)
2. & 3. Dormitories (1848)
4. & 5. Professors' Residence (1848)
6. Chapel (toward's Hall (1848)
7. The Chapel (1853)
8. & 9. Carriage House (1857)
10. Dormitory (1857)

11. New Steward's Hall (1857)
12. The Gymnasium (1857)
13. The Observatory (1859)
14. The Magnetic Observatory (1860)
15. The Path to the Depot
16. The Road to Oxford

Drawing courtesy of Deborah J. Thiel Freeland, Oxford, Miss.

Ole Miss Campus, Oxford, where the Sisters nursed 1,500 Confederate wounded from the Battle of Shiloh. They evacuated 940 men by rail before Grant's forces descended on Oxford.

Buildings 7, the chapel, and 13, the observatory, were used for hospitals; Building 14, the magnetic observatory, was the morgue.

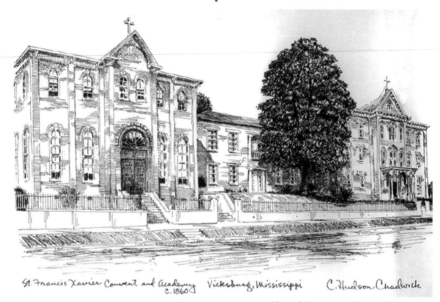

St Francis Xavier Convent and Academy   Vicksburg, Mississippi   C. Hudson Chadwick
C. 1860

Sketch by C. Hudson Chadwick.
Sketch of the building as it stands presently. St. Catherine's is behind the magnolia tree. Now the Southern Heritage Cultural Center.

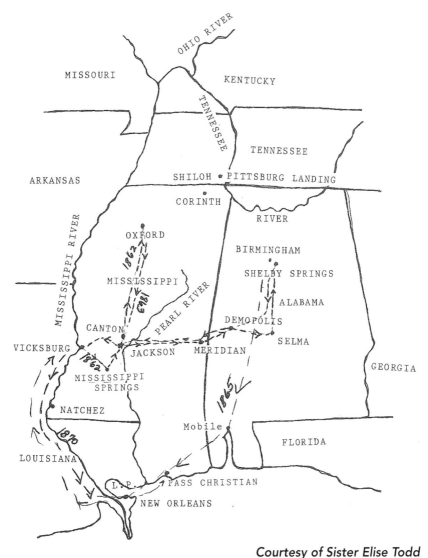

Courtesy of Sister Elise Todd

*Travels of the Sisters during the War: 1862, Vicksburg to Mississippi Springs;
1862 on to Jackson, 1862, on to Oxford; 1863, by rail back to Jackson;
1863, after fall of Vicksburg and Jackson on to Shelby Springs by rail with
wounded; 1864, two return to Vicksburg from Shelby Springs; then four,
then in March 1865, one postulant brought to Jackson to be picked up,
taken to Vicksburg, May 30, 1865 four remaining Sisters and Father Leray
journey back to Vicksburg by way of Mobile and New Orleans taking two
weeks. In 1870, Sisters take steamboat NATCHEZ to New Orleans and
another boat over Lake Pontchartrain to the first branch house
Pass Christian.*

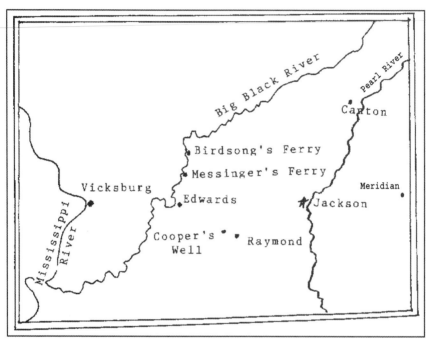

Courtesy of Sister Elise Todd.
The 10-day approximately 50-mile stint from Vicksburg to Jackson taken by
Sister DeSales and John Kearney in horse and buggy in 1864 and 90 more
miles to Meridian. The Big Black River had to be crossed on Messinger's
Ferry; this is the same route taken to get Amanaide Poursine in March 1865
when she is brought to Jackson from Shelby Springs to be received as
Sister Xavier.
Cooper's Well was directly adjacent to Mississippi Springs.

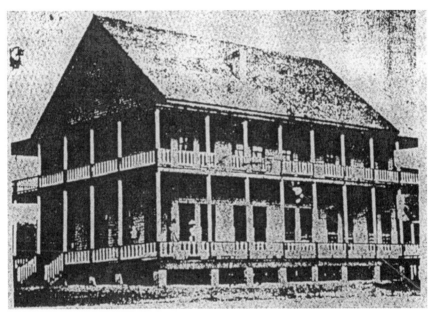

Courtesy Shelby County Historical Society.
The Shelby Springs Resort Building in Alabama used for a hospital by the Sisters.

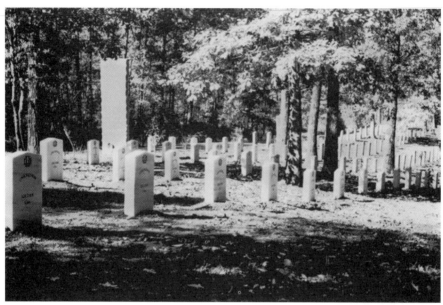

Courtesy Ken Penhale
Site of the recently restored Shelby Springs Cemetery adjacent to the hospital.

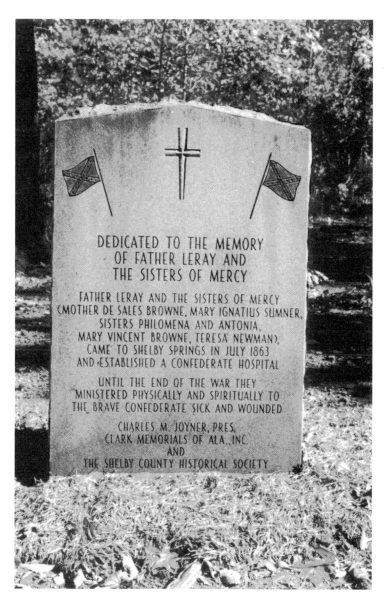

DEDICATED TO THE MEMORY
OF FATHER LERAY AND
THE SISTERS OF MERCY

FATHER LERAY AND THE SISTERS OF MERCY
(MOTHER DE SALES BROWNE, MARY IGNATIUS SUMNER,
SISTERS PHILOMENA AND ANTONIA,
MARY VINCENT BROWNE, TERESA NEWMAN),
CAME TO SHELBY SPRINGS IN JULY 1863
AND ESTABLISHED A CONFEDERATE HOSPITAL

UNTIL THE END OF THE WAR THEY
MINISTERED PHYSICALLY AND SPIRITUALLY TO
THE BRAVE CONFEDERATE SICK AND WOUNDED

CHARLES M. JOYNER, PRES.
CLARK MEMORIALS OF ALA., INC.
AND
THE SHELBY COUNTY HISTORICAL SOCIETY

Courtesy Ken Penhale

*Monument in Shelby Springs Cemetery dedicated to Father
Leray and the Sisters of Mercy.*

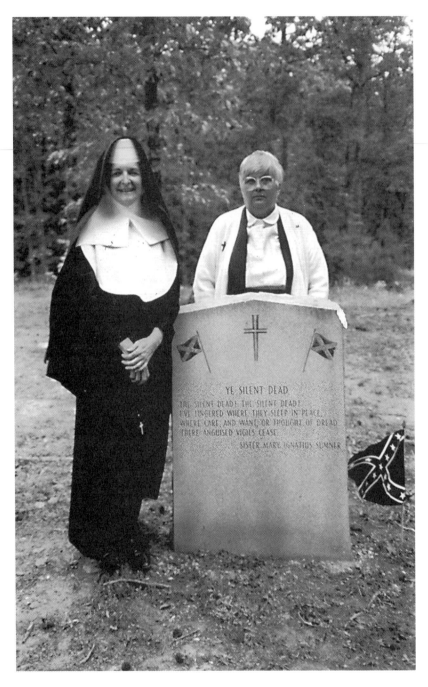

Re-enactment of parts of the Civil War Diary at the annual Shelby Springs Cemetery event. Glenda La Garde as Sister Ignatius, and editor Sister Mary Paulinus.

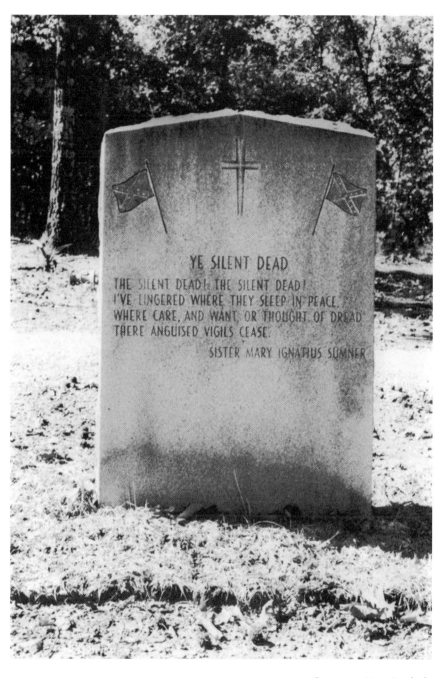

YE SILENT DEAD
THE SILENT DEAD! THE SILENT DEAD!
I'VE LINGERED WHERE THEY SLEEP IN PEACE,
WHERE CARE, AND WANT OR THOUGHT OF DREAD
THERE ANGUISED VIGILS CEASE.

SISTER MARY IGNATIUS SUMNER

Courtesy Ken Penhale

Monument commemorating Sister Ignatius' poem "Ye Silent Dead" at Shelby Springs Cemetery.

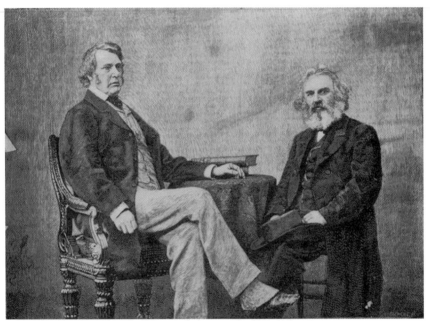

Photograph of Sister Ignatius' uncle, Senator Charles Sumner and Henry Wadsworth Longfellow found in Sister's scrap book.

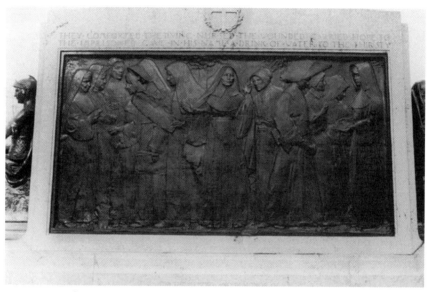

***Washington D.C. Monument reprinted with the permission of the
U.S. Catholic Health Association***

Picture of the monument in Washington, D.C., honoring the Sisters from
the 12 religious communities who served in the Civil War as Sister-nurses.
Sisters pictured on the monument are; Sisters of St. Ursula, Galveston,
Texas; Sisters of Providence, St. Mary of the Woods, Indiana; Sisters of the
Holy Cross, Notre Dame, Indiana; Sisters of Our Lady of Mount Carmel,
New Orleans, Louisiana; Sisters of the Poor of St. Francis, Cincinnati, Ohio;
Sisters of St. Joseph, Philadelphia and Wheeling West Virginia; Sisters of
St. Dominic, Kentucky, Tennessee, and Illinois; Sisters of Charity of Nazareth
Kentucky, Sisters of Charity of New York and Cincinnati, Daughters of Char-
ity Emmitsburg, Maryland; Sisters of Mercy Pittsburgh, New York, Chicago,
Baltimore, Vicksburg, Cincinnati; Sisters of Our Lady of Mercy Charleston,
South Carolina who later affiliated with the Sisters of Mercy.

This information was compiled by Ellen Jolly in the book Nuns of the Battlefield. The author did extensive research and the monument was erected in
1924 by the Ancient Order of Hibernians. Subsequent research attests to
many more communities of sisters who served. This monument is located
at the junction of Rhode Island and Connecticut Avenues across the street
from St. Matthew's Cathedral.

Sister Mary Agnes Maddigan
Sister Mary Philomena Farmer
1842-1876

The two young women from Baltimore, who cast their young lives with the Sisters of Mercy Community bound for the Mississippi Southern Mission, were intricately bound together in life and death as Sisters in religion and ministry. Their roots are rather anonymous as there is no listing of their parents or family backgrounds.

Both young women, each 17 years of age, decided to join the Sisters on this Southern adventure, and little did anyone know what lay ahead for these refined, well educated young women during their wartime travels.

Mary Maddigan came with the four professed Sisters and arrived in Vicksburg in October 1860. Rose Farmer came on her own a few months later and entered the Sisters of Mercy at St. Francis, Vicksburg. Kate Reynolds had come with the original group but was sent home when the war started.[1]

A custom of the foundress, Catherine McAuley, was to send young sisters with each new foundation so that soon after their arrival a public ceremony would be held for all the city to see. So their reception of the White Veil to become novices after being with the Sisters for six months was quite an event in Vicksburg. Their ceremony of initiation into the Sisters of Mercy was described in the local paper:

> *Interesting Ceremony — St. Paul's (Catholic) Church of this city was, yesterday evening, the scene of a very interesting and impressive ceremony, on the occasion of two young ladies taking the White Veil. It was the first scene of the kind ever witnessed in this city. The services were performed by Bishop Elder, of Natchez, assisted by Fathers LeRay, Pont and Elia. There was an immense audience in attendance and the two young ladies Miss Mary Maddigan, and Miss Rose Farmer, who were the candidates for the White Veil, were the center of attraction. They received the religious names of Sister Agnes and Sister Philomena. One of the most striking features of the ceremony was the representations of angels by eight young girls, dressed in appropriate costumes who followed a young girl bearing the silver crucifix while entering the Church.*

> *This is the first degree in initiating these young ladies*
> *into the novitiate of the Sisters of Mercy. The duties of this*
> *religious order of the Catholic Church are a life of mercy*
> *to the needy and distressed, to relieve the wants of the poor,*
> *attend on the sick, and to educate the young. They conse-*
> *crate their services to a life of mercy, of charity and useful-*
> *ness. All who witnessed the ceremony were deeply im-*
> *pressed with the solemnity and appropriateness in which*
> *it was conducted.*[2]

War came, and a year later Vicksburg was heavily shelled. These two young novices began a novitiate unlike any other in the history of the order. After two years of teaching school, they began their nursing pilgrimage all over Mississippi and Alabama. They shared the fears and horrors of the war with the early Sisters. They suffered want and sorrow. They made their vows of total commitment in Vicksburg. Sister Philomena returned to Vicksburg in 1864 with the other three Sisters to reclaim the property and start school. They were trying to establish some degree of normalcy in the city and convent, so with only half of the Sisters present, school was resumed. Sister Philomena was professed at St. Paul's January 6, 1865.[3] Sister Agnes remained in Shelby Springs as a nurse, so she did not profess her vows until after her return in May 1865. In the presence of Bishop Elder, she professed her vows in Vicksburg June 4, 1866[4]. She had been in the community for six years having been received five years before. She had been a postulant in 1860, when the original group came. She had remained in Shelby Springs until the Sisters returned, and peace came May 30, 1865. A number of young ladies had entered as postulants. She served another year in Vicksburg before making her vows. Her youth, shy disposition and traumatic six years in wartime travel may have given her doubts or perhaps the community had doubts as to her suitability, thus the delay. Canon law prescribed a year of deep spiritual preparation which these two young ladies had constantly interrupted by war, travels, and travails. Agnes particularly is lauded for her spirit of prayer. Mixing the active and spiritual life was a hallmark of the Mercy Sisters, but Sisters Philomena and Agnes' novitiate certainly emphasized the active.

Returning to St. Francis, working to restore the ravaged buildings both resumed teaching and visitation. Sister Philomena was particularly successful in teaching the boys. The Sisters had begun to teach night school to men, who desired to further their education. One John Loviza, river boat captain, builder of river boats, owner of the first coal yard in Vicksburg, was one of the first night students. He, as a very young man, wrecked the tugboat, "Thistle," at the foot of Clay Street.

After this episode, he went back to working in the family store and began night school. This must have been around 1868 or 1869. He wrote in later years: "Among those who taught me at night school were Sister Antonia, Sister Philomena and Sister Xavier and I feel sure that they are all in heaven for they surely were good to me."[5]

Sister Agnes seemed to be a shy, quiet person. The annals mention "She had frail health which was caused by the rigors of War and a severe spell of typhoid fever which left her a silent sufferer for years." She was known for her great simplicity of character and her spirit of prayer.[6]

Sister Philomena was sent on the first branch house mission with Sister Mary Vincent to Pass Christian in 1870 and remained there for some time. In early 1876 she was there, when the church burned. Father Henry Georget, the French priest Father Leray had brought from France in 1857, was the Sisters' pastor and friend. This was probably her last traumatic event before her death in late 1876.

The obituary book says, "Sister was a successful teacher and will be remembered for making many visitations to the sick and shut-ins."[7]

Both young Sisters were in Vicksburg in late 1876. Sister Agnes had been nursing Sister Philomena who was dying the slow lingering last days of consumption. Sister Agnes, always rather frail and delicate, had walking pneumonia and died very suddenly in October, so suddenly that the priest was not summoned in time for the last rites.

Deeply saddened by the death of her dearest friend and nurse, Sister Philomena died in December, 1876. Her reception of the last rites, her wake and funeral services were most dramatic in a city that loved this young woman and so keenly felt her loss.

Both Sister Philomena and Sister Agnes had entered the Sisters of Mercy at age 17. Both had given their all for seventeen years. The first to be buried in the Convent Cemetery at St. Francis were the first to enter. Both were interred at the age of 34.

A newspaper tribute applies to both Sisters equally well:

> *...Seventeen years of beautiful labor — visiting the sick and afflicted and administering to their wants. During the late war they exposed themselves to many dangers in attending the sick and wounded and regardless of their own welfares, they were mindful of promoting the happiness of others.*[8]

One of Sister Philomena's boys wrote a tribute to her in the paper:

*...The writer knew her for years, and to her he is indebted
for many of the happiest moments of his life. Her gentle
and amiable disposition won the hearts of all who knew
her, and left impressions too endearing to be forgotten soon.
A solemn Mass of Requiem was said on Monday at 8
o'clock [Death Dec. 17, 1876] and afterwards her remains
were borne, by her former students, to their final resting
place.*
*...Fervent were the prayers which they offered that she who
loved them on earth would not forget them in heaven.*
   *May thy slumbers be quiet and peaceful, may the angels
and bright choirs of heavens be thy companions! and may
thy pure soul enjoy the sweet embrace of Him whom thou
has served so long, is the fervent prayer of an old pupil.*

A soul like hers, so high and pure,
This sinful world could not allure;
It longed to break the heavy chain
Which bound it to a mortal shell,
And soar aloft to Heaven's domain,
With God and blessed souls to dwell,
And in the essence of His love
Dissolve itself with Him above.

Tossed over life's tempestuous sea.
Look down on us from thy bright shrine;
Pray that our last end may be
As holy and as calm as thine.[9]
                    T.A.G.

Sister Stephana Warde
1829 (?) - 1904

The story of Anne Warde, cousin of the American foundress Mother Xavier Warde, has to be the most colorful and enigmatic of the original group of Sisters in Vicksburg. Irish-born Anne came to Pittsburgh with her family, entered the Sisters of Mercy in 1849 and took the name of Sister Stephana.[1] She went to Baltimore in 1855 with Sister DeSales and the original group who took over the Washington Infirmary, in its incipient stages. She nursed there for five years efficiently and compassionately until she volunteered to go to the Vicksburg mission with the pioneer group. She was a lay sister who kept house and instructed girls in home management and serving.

Sister Ignatius mentions her by name in the first part of the journal as one of the original sisters. She is never mentioned again in the journal or the annals of the Sisters.

Her story from there is from her own accounts related to the Sisters in Pittsburgh where she allegedly returned after the War (she actually nursed at the Stanton Hospital in 1865 for a few months). Although she came from the Baltimore foundation, she had entered and made her religious profession in Pittsburgh, so she had the privilege to return to Pittsburgh if she wished. This account is given in the *History of Pittsburgh Mercy Hospital 1847-1899* from the Pittsburgh Archives:

> *The Sisters left Vicksburg with the other evacuees and nursed their patients in camps, barns, abandoned railroad stations or in army tents around Oxford, Mississippi Springs, Jackson and Shelby Springs, Alabama. The Sisters' chaplain contrived to visit the various camps whenever the Sisters were there in order to give them the consolation of hearing Mass and receiving the Sacraments.*
>
> *They did little services for him in return, but he was able to look after their physical well-being and even contrived to make them shoes out of rabbit skins when theirs were worn out. Despite the lack even of necessities, often the Sisters and the nursing corps did heroic work for the wounded on both sides sheltering them wherever they could from the rays of a blistering sun, the chill of wintery winds, or from drenching rains.*

Finally Sister Stephana's contingent was captured
by the Union forces. A prisoner-of-war, she had an over-
whelming desire — to get back to Pittsburgh, the convent
of her profession. Sick at heart, her veil tattered, her habit
frayed and worn, she waited for her release. It came in
mid-winter. Dressed in an army coat of the pattern worn
by the Union nurses, she came to Pittsburgh. Arriving one
evening in the city she went straight to St. Mary Convent
on Webster Avenue. It had been twelve years since Sis-
ter had left St. Mary Convent; there was another Sister
Stephana in the Pittsburgh Community in 1865. When a
Sister opened the door, she was startled at the haggard
looking woman standing there in a partial Union uniform.
She welcomed the stranger and went for the superior. She
too was startled by the wearing apparel, the absence of
coif and gimp and the religious habit. She served Sister
Stephana some supper and listened to her story. Finally,
Sister Stephana put her hand to her throat, pulled out a
soiled bag, broke the string and produced her vows which
she had carried over her heart since leaving Vicksburg.

She was weary and ill but asked to be reinstated in the
community, and after her recovery in the hospital for a
short time, she went down to Stanton Hospital to help the
Sisters there. A Corps of Pittsburgh Mercies nursed in long
rows of frame buildings named for Secretary of War. Sol-
diers from the front were brought there. The Sisters shifted
Sister nurses from Pittsburgh.[2]

Her name does not appear on the muster rolls of the War Department for that hospital. Nor was she included in the list of those who
served at Vicksburg. After her short stint of nursing in the Stanton
Hospital, the Sisters were withdrawn after the War. She spent her last
years at Mercy Hospital in Pittsburgh where she often recounted her
war experiences. She celebrated her golden jubilee at St. Mary Convent,
Webster Avenue, December 18, 1901; she died November 4, 1904 and is
buried at St. Xavier Cemetery Latrobe, Pennsylvania.[3]

There are some mysteries in her story. She returned a few
months before the war ended. In *Nuns of the Battlefield* by Ellen
Jolly, 1927, it is stated: "In after years, Sister Stephana often said
with a smile that for this double duty, she had been doubly rewarded

in this world, upon the evening she met President Lincoln upon the occasion of his first visit to the Stanton Hospital Washington, D.C."[4]

The silence of the Vicksburg community is rather overwhelming in Sister Stephana's regard. Why did she leave? Sister Healy's biography of Sister Francis Warde does tell us that she had relatives fighting for the Union.[5] She had been nursing both Confederate and Union wounded for three years. When exactly did she leave? In her own oral account she claimed to have left with a military escort. Where was she captured? Why is there no written account in the very thorough journal and archives? Why are there no letters or references made to letters? She must have nursed at Shelby Springs up until the time that the four Sisters returned to Vicksburg to reclaim the property since several sources record that there were eight Sisters there. The four who went to Vicksburg and left Shelby Spring were Sisters DeSales, Ignatius, Margaret Ferrens (Sr. Antonia), and Rose Farmer (Sister Philomena). The four who remained at Shelby Springs were Sister Vincent, Teresa Newman, Agnes Maddigan and Stephana Ward. Sister Ignatius would not have been there to record her departure. The four left Shelby Springs May 23, 1864; the property in Vicksburg was restored July 25, 1864.[6] There is nothing written about Sister Stephana. Only in eternity will the whole story of this Sister of Mercy be revealed.

Sister Teresa Newman
1823-1895

Martha Newman was the first young lady from Vicksburg to become a Sister of Mercy. According to Mother Bernard's accounts, she entered the community March 2, in 1861, fourteen months previous to the opening naval bombardment of the city. She received the religious habit September 5, 1861 at "St. Paul's Church which was elaborately decorated and crowded to the utmost, since all were desirous of witnessing a ceremony so new in a city still full of members of the 'Know-Nothing Society.' " All were deeply impressed with the beauty and solemnity of the occasion. For the first time, perhaps they vaguely understood the heroism of the sacrifice made."[1] Two postulants, Mary Maddigan and Rose Farmer from Baltimore, had been received at St. Paul's April 8, 1861, only five months previously with great attention from the local congregation. Martha Newman was a convert to Catholicism and a member of an old and well-established family in Vicksburg. She had been educated in Kentucky at the Charity Sisters' Academy which many of the non-Catholic Southern young ladies attended because of its reputation for a fine education.[2] She was a popular, mature lady of the Vicksburg community, being thirty-eight at the time of her reception. Many non-Catholics must have attended the ceremony at which time she received the name Sister Teresa. She lived a dedicated life as a Sister of Mercy living through some historical events; she was a well-read person, and her knowledge of historical events was phenomenal. She had the happiness of serving the community in every capacity, according to Mother Bernard.

She made her vows at Shelby Springs. Sisters Philomena and Agnes, the first postulants, made their profession much later. She was the only one to do so, probably because of her age and fear of death. Being a mature person and having the desire to dedicate herself totally, she made her profession on a makeshift altar on a cold January morning in 1863 with sycamore balls burning in lard oil for lights instead of candles. What a contrast to her reception at St. Paul's Church with all its elegance.[3] She cherished this memory and shared with all the newly professed this dramatic story of her wartime profession.

What a morale boost this must have been at this time! At this period in history the code of canon law had not developed to allow Sisters to take temporary vows for a time before final vows. The first vows were for life.

Actually Sister Teresa was slightly older than both Sister DeSales and Sister Ignatius. This Vicksburger from one of the oldest, most prosperous families returned to her "hill city" in 1865, with rabbit-skin shoes and tattered black clothing sewed with white thread.

She served 34 years in the community. Mother Bernard's book says she lived many long and useful years:

> *She was a popular story teller among the young sisters recounting the events of hardships and privations during the "Confederacy." She was an example throughout her life of practicing habits of rigorous poverty and self denial which she learned from necessity during the war years.*[4]

Sister Mary Xavier Poursine
1842-1918

Although this Sister did not come from Baltimore, she is one of the pioneer band who entered on the battlefield, as it were, of the Civil War and epitomized all a Sister of Mercy should be until her death in 1918.

Aminaide was from a French Creole family from New Orleans. Her father, Pierre Poursine, had been a great benefactor and fellow worker with the Jesuit priests in that city. General Benjamin Butler had occupied New Orleans in the spring of 1862 and was extremely offensive to those loyal to the Confederacy there. He forced them to take a loyalty oath or suffer dire consequences. He confiscated the home of the Poursines, and they were forced to leave New Orleans.

A number of exiled Creole families had taken up temporary residence in a little town in Alabama named Cahaba. This was near the resort Shelby Springs. When the Sisters arrived there in 1863, with their trainload of refugee wounded, the Poursines were very happy to see them. Pierre Poursine and Father LeRay conversed in French. The entire family became friendly and helpful to the Sisters. Aminaide joined in helping the Sisters nurse at the hospital. She had to wait until the Sisters returned to Vicksburg for her reception. She entered officially December 18, 1864, and was received April 6, 1865, in Vicksburg. Toward the end of the war Sister Mary Vincent and Father Leray brought her to Jackson where she was met by Sister DeSales to return to Vicksburg. Four Sisters remained in Shelby Springs; four resumed classes in Vicksburg. Aminaide made the fifth. Later her younger sister, Amelie, entered and became Sister Stanislaus.[1]

Amelie Poursine was an introvert. She worked laboriously in the City Hospital for its duration and died in 1912. She was known among the Sisters for being a dedicated religious and for practicing the hidden virtues and performing obscure duties.

Sister Bernard's book gives some sketchy information about the family, but she does tell that Aminaide's mother was the great-granddaughter of a distinguished French family, who had suffered in the massacre of slaves in Santo Domingo. Her great-grandmother was rescued by a slave who escaped in a tiny boat. The boat capsized before they reached land, but the two were saved by the crew of a sailing vessel.[2]

The Poursine daughters Aminaide, Amelie, and Melanie were reared in the French Quarter of New Orleans and educated at the thriving convent school at Convent, Louisiana where hundreds of young New Orleans girls took a boat up the Mississippi River for their education. This school flourished before Sacred Heart Academy on St. Charles Avenue and was run by the Religious of the Sacred Heart.

Aminaide was a selfless Christian young lady from the beginning. Although from a wealthy family, she had been brought up with great sensitivity to the poor and suffering. The wounded soldiers appreciated her gentle ministrations and vivacious enthusiasm.[3]

She nursed through the yellow fever epidemics. Unfortunately no letters remain from her mother and three aunts who were Religious of the Sacred Heart. Eighteen of their nuns died at the Baton Rouge Foundation from the 1878 fever, probably former teachers of Aminaide and her sisters.[4]

Her ministry in Vicksburg was dedicated to education and to the poor. Her unfailing devotion to God's poor was an outstanding characteristic. Long before there were any charitable associations or community chests in the parish, she organized among her former pupils a society for the aid of the poor. She had an office and two store rooms of clothes and groceries. Numerous needy ones received aid from this well managed department.[5]

She had a reliable Black assistant, Leanna. Both were extremely sensitive to the feelings of the recipients. Sister would say, "I will not have my poor criticized by unfeeling strangers." They constructed a curious lattice work arrangement where the poor could come and go with their baskets almost unseen.[6]

It seems that for many years she prepared the First Communion classes. She also served many years as Reverend Mother of the Community.

Home visitation was one of Sister Xavier's hallmarks; she visited mothers with newborns and often suggested names for many of them. At the other end of the spectrum, she prayed with the dying.

The newspaper obituaries tell much of the impact of the deceased on the local community. One headline SISTER M. XAVIER STILL REMEMBERED BY HER "CHILDREN" — UNFAILING DEVOTION TO GOD'S POOR FOREVER SHOWN.

Excerpts from the obituary:

> *Sister Xavier, familiarly known as the "Angel of Mercy," was beloved by all, irrespective of creed or denomination for she recognized neither of these in her beneficent good deeds for humanity. Her life was a beautiful one of self-immolation....She celebrated her golden jubilee in which all of Vicksburg participated with much happiness....A gentle spirit has passed, and her good deeds live with the generations left. She was truly a part of Vicksburg's history, and her passing leaves a void...[7]*

Father Francis Xavier Leray
1825-1887

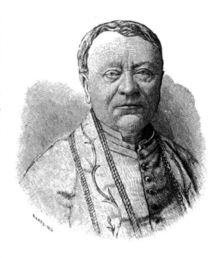

Francis Leray was born in a small town near Rennes, France, in 1825. His family were people of means. He always had money and returned often to France. As a young man he came to a very pluralistic society. It is interesting that he left France, just before the height of Napoleon's conquests, to come to Mississippi, the heart of the Protestant Bible Belt mentality. The Eudist Fathers had been his teachers in France. He began his studies in Spring Hill College in Mobile, Alabama, in 1845; he entered St. Mary's Seminary in Baltimore in 1847; he was accepted as a student for the Diocese of Natchez in 1850. In 1851, he accompanied some of the Eudist priests to Natchez to teach at the college the bishop had recently established there, which failed after two years. In 1852, he started his ministry in the diocese where he was one of only seven priests under Bishop James Van de Velde. The Catholic population areas were the three towns of Natchez, Vicksburg and Jackson, with pockets of Catholics in Yazoo City, Canton, Sulphur Springs, and the Gulf Coast. The bishop took horseback tours of the sweeping diocese, but each priest also had large parish territories to cover to reach the sparse Catholic population. Leray was pastor of St. Peter's Jackson from 1852-57 and also served in Canton 30 miles away. Serving this capital city area and its surroundings comprised a great expanse of territory.[1]

While serving at St. Peter's, Jackson, Leray started the first Catholic school there with John Kelly as instructor. Kelly was the father of Sister Bonaventure Kelly, who entered the Mercy community in 1885. The school consisted of forty pupils, twenty-five of whom were Catholic. Leray completed the rectory and purchased the bell and organ. He purchased Father John Baptist Babonneau's chalice to be his while in the diocese but afterwards to revert to the diocese. Father Babonneau, a young priest, was his predecessor and had died of yellow fever before Leray became pastor. Leray served in Jackson during the yellow fever epidemics of 1852, '54, '55 and in Vicksburg during the 1878 epidemic. Many Mississippians died as did a number of his fellow priests. He was sick with the fever in 1878 but was one of the few priests to survive. A priority among the clergy during the epidemics and war was to be there to administer the last sacraments to dying Catholics. He was a fervent, dedicated priest who always took this ministry seriously.[2]

An astute business man, a motivator, a lover of education, Leray was always devoted to his people. In 1857 he returned to France to seek priests for the diocese. When he arrived there, he found his mother had died. This left him in a state of depression. However, in a short time, he returned to Mississippi with Father Henry Georget. This priest served as a devoted pastor and exemplary priest on the Gulf Coast and was pastor and friend to the Sisters on their first branch house in Pass Christian, Mississippi.[3]

An interesting incident is recorded in the letters to Bishop Elder indicating the scrupulosity of Father Leray. In 1858 General James Quitman, former governor and Mexican War hero, was to be buried in a Protestant church.[4] Father Leray felt his civic duty to attend but asked permission of Bishop Elder who in his characteristic manner encouraged Leray to let his conscience be his guide.[5]

In 1859, he was made pastor of St. Paul's Vicksburg replacing Father Jeremiah O'Connor, who had purchased a two-story house for a school, anticipating that Sisters would come. Typical of the solicitude he, as well as the Bishop, had for Catholics in the area, Bishop Elder requested him to visit Millikens Bend on the river on the Louisiana side, about fifty miles by horseback. The bishop had heard that there was sickness there. Leray had concern over the large number of poor immigrant children living in shanties on or close to the levee in Vicksburg and was most anxious to have the school started. In 1860, he went to Baltimore to accompany the Sisters of Mercy to Vicksburg. Sister DeSales, the leader of the group, was a docile, rather timid person, although she always acted according to her convictions. She and Father Leray seemed to complement each other from the beginning of the ministry. Both were quick to respond to the needs of the most downtrodden. He was protective of the Sisters and it was noted in Sister Ignatius journal that he made shoes for the Sisters from rabbit skins at Shelby Springs toward the end of the Civil War. In a very early incident when the school had opened, the affluent neighbors protested the shanty boat Irish children bringing down the neighborhood by their very presence. The diplomat,

Father Leray dispelled their fears and assured them that the Sisters were capable of handling the situation. He prudently added that the large arbor vitae bushes would shelter their view. In dealing with dying soldiers, his straightforward manner and sometimes abrasive attitude, especially toward Protestant ministers, contrasted sharply with the more gentle, ecumenical style of the Sisters. There is never a critical word in any of the Vicksburg annals about Father Leray.[6]

At the outbreak of the war, Bishop Elder had only twelve priests, and he encouraged them to serve as civilian chaplains where they were needed, since he did not want his congregations devoid of the sacraments. Father Rene Pont, a young priest, enlisted and received a commission at the beginning of the war and took the Bishop by surprise. The Bishop did not like to have the priests seek or accept commissions as official Confederate chaplains; as civilian chaplains they could move freely among units and could leave without difficulty. It seemed that Father Leray was a civilian chaplain during the war. By the end of the conflict, seven priests had served as full time chaplains; four others as part time. Four died because of the war. The Vicar General of the diocese, Father Mathurin Grignon was partly crippled and was not able to serve on the missions, and no mention is made of his serving in the war.[7]

Leray was with the Sisters in many of their journeys during most of the war. He was chaplain at Oxford and sent for the Sisters from Jackson. He was with them and the wounded in Jackson before and during the siege of Vicksburg; he accompanied them to Shelby Springs and was there the last year of the war. He appeared in other places without the Sisters, e.g., Holly Springs 1862, Battle of Raymond 1863. In 1864 he was at Shelby Springs, Alabama, and he reported to Bishop Elder for directions. His choices as he presented them to Elder were to join troops in the field as chaplain, stay with the hospital work or return to Vicksburg. Returning to Vicksburg seemed least wise since the military authorities intended to deal harshly with all clergymen who had actively supported the rebellion. The Bishop himself had suffered reprisals from the commander in Natchez and was banished for a time to Vidalia, Louisiana. The bishop advised him to stay at Shelby Springs since General Henry Slocum would not let him enter Vicksburg with the Sisters. Slocum said, "What! Let Father Leray enter? I would as soon let in one of Forrest's brigades."[8]

Father Leray was outspoken in his loyalty to the Confederacy. Both he and Bishop Elder had special Masses at Vicksburg, in St. Paul's and the Natchez Cathedral when local units left around Christmas in 1861.

A high Mass was held where the entire company with arms attended. Father Leray blessed the flag of the "Jeff Davis Guards," a predominantly Irish unit. The ceremony was described as "a novel spectacle for the Protestants." In October of 1861, Father Charles Heuze was sent to Vicksburg as assistant. He served there during Leray's absence. An Irish priest, Father Patrick McCabe, came as an assistant in 1864. He arrived about the time that four of the Sisters had returned from Shelby Springs to reclaim and restart the school. Father McCabe helped with the teaching and served until his untimely death from typhoid only eight months later.[9]

It is noted in the Bishop's writings that Leray suffered from facial paralysis in 1870; this must have been temporary. In the diocesan archives, there are records of his periodically donating money to the orphanage in Natchez, another of his favorite causes. There is also record of Bishop Elder borrowing $4,000 from him. In 1867, Leray lent money to the Sisters to build an addition to the convent and school. He did not ask for repayment of the money, $4,000, until he was raised to the episcopacy. He became Bishop of Natchitoches, Louisiana in 1877. This was a diocese with over 25,000 Catholics, twice the size of the Mississippi diocese in population, but in an extremely poor section of the country. This is presently the diocese of Alexandria, Louisiana.[10] Ironically the Religious of the Sacred Heart from Louisiana had opened a school there in 1847 but had to close it in 1851.

From this time forward, Leray was beset with financial problems in his area of ministry. The Mercy Sisters in his new diocese had a foundation from the New Orleans group. Because of the poverty of the place, they were unable to survive; he disbanded them and sent one fine professed Sister, Sister Josephine Trichell, a native of Natchitoches, along with a retarded woman for whom the Sisters had cared, to the Vicksburg community. Sister DeSales accepted both in her hospitable, gracious manner. The other Sisters returned to New Orleans from where they had originally come. Sister Josephine spent the greater part of her life serving the sick at City Hospital in Vicksburg. She was a skilled nurse familiar with the "old creole" remedies.[11]

Leray remained administrator of Natchitoches until 1883 although he had been named coadjutor of New Orleans in 1879. As ordinary of New Orleans, his chief concern was the reduction of his predecessor's debts in a nearly bankrupted diocese. This he attempted from 1883 until his death in 1887. He was unpopular in the area following the dearly loved Archbishop Napoleon Perche and strapped with the financial pressures of his office. These factors probably brought on his death at age 62.[12]

There are a series of letters, most in the New Orleans archdiocesan archives, from Sister DeSales from 1879-1887 until Leray's death, showing she sent him small amounts of money. There is one letter obtained from the New Orleans archives to Sister DeSales from Leray. It is dated 1879; he requested payment of the $4,000 that had been borrowed 12 years previously and asked that $400 be paid a year for as long as he lived and at the time of his death the $4,000 principal would revert back to the Sisters. Sister DeSales sent him small amounts periodically. Several accounts indicate that in 1887 the $4,000 had been paid to the penny. The new archbishop of New Orleans, Jannsens, who was from Mississippi, told the Sisters they had paid sufficiently.[13] There is nothing recorded in the Vicksburg archives to indicate that the Sisters were willed anything by Leray. He died in France on a visit there in 1887 and was buried there. Very few facts were listed about him in the *Catholic Encyclopedia;* Sister Ignatius' *Journal* depicted him as a friend and protector of the Sisters. He is described from Mother Bernard's book by those who knew him as "a blunt and determined man," "distant" and "aloof"; he was also known as a "most capable administrator," and "a man of profound faith and piety."[14]

His dedication as a chaplain was unparalleled. Of the twenty-eight priests who served as Confederate chaplains, Leray was one of three who was raised to the episcopacy, the other two being Dominic Manucy, Mobile, and Anthony Pellicer, San Antonio.[15]

Endnotes

Sister Ignatius Sumner

[1]Sister Austin Carroll, *Leaves from the Annals of the Sisters of Mercy*, Vol. IV, 76.

[2]Baltimore Mercy Archives.

[3]Mother M. Bernard Maguire, R.S.M., *The Story of the Sisters of Mercy in Mississippi,* 42.

[4]Georgetown University Archives and *Woodstock Letters*, a Jesuit publication of Woodstock College, obituaries and information on the Sumner brothers.

[5]Thomas W. Higginson, *Margaret Fuller Ossoli,* 92.

[6]Special Collections: Lauinger Library, Georgetown University, Washington, D.C., information, and obituaries on Sumner brothers.

[7]Archives of Loyola College in Baltimore, Maryland, information on Sumner brothers and family records.

[8]Special Collections.

[9]Ibid.

[10]Vicksburg, Mississippi Archives of the Sisters of Mercy, Annals, chronicles, notes, original letters and documents, recollections of senior Sisters, twenty scrapbooks, minutes of meetings, funeral home records, newspaper clippings, obituaries, Sister Ignatius Sumner's personal scrapbook, the original manuscript of the journal and the expanded journal done from dictation before Sister Ignatius died, other journals the *Choctaw Mission Journal* by Sister Marcelline Street, the *Edwards Yellow Fever Journal* by Sister Angela Fedou, five manuscripts.

[11]Ibid.

[12]Ibid, from scrapbook unidentified newspaper article.

[13]Ibid.

[14]Mother M. Bernard, 216.

[15]Vicksburg Mercy Archives.

[16]David H. Donald, *Charles Sumner and the Coming of the Civil War*, 8.

[17]Special Collections.

[18]Baltimore Mercy Archives.

[19]Memoirs of the Pittsburgh Sisters of Mercy 1843-1917, 65

[20]Baltimore Mercy Archives.

[21]Mother M. Bernard, 43.

[22]Sister M. Loretto Costello, *Sisters of Mercy of Maryland 1855-1930*, 13-16.

[23]Sister Austin Carroll, Vol. IV, 67.

[24]Sister M. Loretto, 36.

[25]Mother M. Bernard, 49.

> Ye Silent Dead!
> The silent dead. 'The silent dead.'
> I've lingered where they sleep in peace,
> Where care, and want, or thought of dread
> There anguished vigils cease.

Our silent dead! Our silent dead!
They lure me to their mossy rest,
Where roses, snowy petals shed,
And birds sing requiems in their nest.

O silent dead! O silent dead!
Thus dreams my soul of deathless lands.
For in the limit of your bed
Time and eternity clasp hands.

Ye silent dead! Ye silent dead!
For me to come, for you 'tis passed,
And while the heavens bend o'er your bed
Your lessons wise and holy last.

Then silent dead! O silent dead!
Why should my restless spirit moan?
Your footsteps have to Calvary led,
And thither must my soul be borne.

The peace ye breathe e'en now must come
When the night of time has fled,
When the Bridegroom calls me home
And I too, sleep with the silent dead.

[26]Ibid, 215.

[27]*Vicksburg Evening Post,* June 17, 1895.

[28]Vicksburg Mercy Archives.

[29]Ibid.

[30]*Vicksburg Evening Post,* June 17, 1895, obituary.

Sister Mary DeSales Browne
[1]Mother M. Bernard, 4.

[2]Ibid.

[3]Buffalo New York Mercy Archives.

[4]Sister Ethelbert Demuth Thesis: *Thy Mercies Will I Sing, History of the Sisters of Mercy, 1860-1960.* Oral interview of Sister Scholastica Gilfoil, June 18, 1960.

[5]Ellen Ryan Jolly, *Nuns of the Battlefield*, 265.

[6]Sister M. Loretto, 3 and 36.

[7]Mother M. Bernard, 8.

[8]Ibid, 13.

[9]Bishop Elder's *Diary*.

[10]Mother M. Bernard, 79.

[11]Vicksburg Mercy Archives.

[12]Court Martial Record, Case Files 1809 - 1938, File No. MM2079, Major General N. J. T. Dana.

[13]Sister Austin Carroll, Volume IV, 366.

[14]Ibid, 368.

[15]Sister Ethelbert, 14.

[16]Sister Austin Carroll, 79.

[17]Mother M. Bernard, 88.

[18]Archives of Diocese of Natchez — Jackson and Vicksburg Mercy Archives.

[19]Archives of Archdiocese of New Orleans.

[20]*Vicksburg Daily Herald* newspaper article from scrapbook undated, approximately April 11, 1898, Vicksburg Mercy Archives.

[21]Mother M. Bernard, 168.

[22]Sister Ethelbert, from an oral interview in 1960 with Sister Loyola Crahen whose father was an assistant roadmaster in 1905.

[23]*Vicksburg Daily Herald* newspaper article from a scrapbook undated, approximately April 14, 1898, title of article: "Eloquent Tribute."

Sister Mary Vincent Brown
[1]Mother M. Bernard, 51.

[2]Sister M. Loretto, 27.

[3]*Vicksburg Weekly Whig* newspaper article, October 27, 1860.

[4]Mother M. Bernard, 53 and 54.

[5]*Vicksburg Evening Post*, September 7, 1937, article by Marie Kearney Lee. The same paper, page 20, by J. Lawrence Gilbert lists some of the first pupils. "The following names of a number of the first pupils of St. Francis Xavier Academy were often told to her children by my mother, Mrs. Cecelia Graf Gilbert, who attended this school on its opening day: Mrs. James Botto, Mrs. K. Benson, Mrs. W. H. Bruser, Mrs. Elizabeth Crofton, Mrs. Tillie Clinton, Mrs. Margaret Smarr David, Mrs. George Doll, Mrs. Fleckenstein, Mrs. Garretty, Mrs. Julia Quinn Geary (the first graduate), Mrs. G. W. Hutcheson, Mrs. Hartman, Mrs. A. L. Jaquith, Mrs. Frank Little, Mrs. John Lavins, Mrs. Josephine Donovan McNamara, Mrs. R. O'Leary, Mrs. A. C. Peatross, Mrs. Margaret Pervangher, Mrs. Kate Ryan, Mrs. J. Voeinkle, Mrs. James Walsh, Miss U. Eunice Orr, Miss Sallie Futrell, Miss Nagle, Miss Cummings. Among the male pupils were James Farrell, John Kearney and William Trowbridge." Bruser's decendants are the Marlettes; Little's, the Hosemans; Voeinkle's, the Yostes.

[6]Mother M. Bernard, 55.

[7]Ibid., 57.

[8]Vicksburg Mercy Archives.

[9]Ibid.

[10]Ibid.

[11]Ibid.

[12]Mother M. Bernard, 61 and 98.

[13]Vicksburg Mercy Archives.

[14]Ibid.

[15]Obituary Scrapbook.

Sister Mary Agnes Maddigan

Sister Mary Philomena Farmer

[1]Sister M. Loretto, 27.

[2]*Vicksburg Evening Citizen* newspaper, April 9, 1861.

[3]Vicksburg Mercy Archives.

[4]Ibid.

[5]*Vicksburg Evening Post* newspaper, December 10, 1989 letter to Post, March 30, 1929 from John Loviza. He was the great grandfather of Joe Loviza elected mayor of Vicksburg in 1993. He was born in Italy in 1850 and died in Vicksburg in 1935.

[6]Vicksburg Mercy Archives.

[7]Obituary Scrapbook.

[8]Vicksburg Mercy Archives. Unidentified newspaper clipping from a scrapbook.

[9]*Vicksburg Herald* unidentified newspaper clipping from scrapbook, approximately December 17, 1876 since that was death date.

Sister Stephana Warde

[1]Pittsburgh Mercy Archives

[2]Ibid.

[3]Ibid.

[4]Ellen Jolly, CCD, *Nuns of the Battlefield*, 121.

[5]Sister Kathleen Healy, RSM, *Frances Warde American Founder of the Sisters of Mercy*, 297.

[6]Vicksburg Mercy Archives.

Sister Teresa Newman

[1]Mother M. Bernard, 10.

[2]Ibid, 11.

[3]Ibid, 11.

[4]Ibid, 11.

Sister Mary Xavier Poursine

[1]Vicksburg Mercy Archives.

[2]Mother M. Bernard, 259.

[3]Ibid, 138.

[4]*Legacy of a Century,* by Sally Reeves, a recently published history of the Religious of the Sacred Heart in Louisiana, identifies three aunts of the Poursine's, blood sisters of their mother, as members of the New Orleans Community. Their last name was Zeringue as was their mother's maiden name.

Melanie was identified as a great benefactor. She became Melanie Poursine Jourdan of Gentilly Plantation.

[5]*Vicksburg Evening Post* newspaper, September 7, 1918.

[6]Mother M. Bernard, 138-143

[7]*Vicksburg Evening Post.*

Francis Xavier Leray

[1]James Pillar, OMI, *The Catholic Church in Mississippi,* 1837-1965, 31.

[2]Vicksburg Mercy Archives.

[3]Mother M. Bernard, 186.

[4]Richard Aubrey McLemore, *A History of Mississippi,* Vol. I, 342.

[5]Archives of Diocese of Jackson, Mississippi.

[6]Vicksburg Mercy Archives.

[7]Pillar, 225-228.

[8]Archives of Diocese – Elder files.

[9]Pillar, 189.

[10]*New Catholic Encyclopedia* Vol. I, 303.

[11]Mother M. Bernard, 264.

[12]*New Catholic Encyclopedia* Vol. I, 303.

[13]Archives of New Orleans – 1879, letters to Sister DeSales.

[14]Mother M. Bernard, 175.

[15]Pillar, 197.

BIBLIOGRAPHY

BOOKS AND PERIODICALS

Barton, George, *Angels of the Battlefield*, 2nd edition, Revised & enlarged. *A History of the Labors of the Catholic Sisterhoods in the Late Civil War.* Philadelphia: The Catholic Art Publishing Co., 1898.

Carrigan, Jo Ann, *The Saffron Scourge, History of Yellow Fever in Louisiana 1796-1905.* Center for Louisiana Studies University of Southwestern Louisiana, Lafayette, Louisiana, 1994.

Carroll, Sister M. Teresa Austin, *Leaves from the Annals of the Sisters of Mercy,* Vols. I, II, III, & IV, New York: P. O'Shea, Publisher, 1895.

College Journal Georgetown College, Dec. 1880. Obituary-student article on John Sumner, founder of the Journal.

Costello, Sister M. Loretto, *Sisters of Mercy of Maryland 1855-1930.* St. Louis: B. Herder Book Co. 1931.

Cotton, Gordon, *The Murder of Minerva Cook*, Gordon Cotton, Vicksburg, Mississippi, 1993.

Demuth, Sister Elizabeth Jean, RSM. Thesis: *Thy Mercies Will I Sing. History of Sisters of Mercy from 1860-1960.* Summaries of Oral Interviews.

Donald, David H. *Charles Sumner and the Coming of the Civil War.* New York: Knopf, 1960.

Donald, David H. *Charles Sumner and the Rights of Man.* New York: Knopf, 1970.

Elder, Bishop William Henry, Bishop of Natchez, *Civil War Diary 1862-1865*. Natchez: Most Rev. R. O. Gerow, Bishop of Natchez-Jackson.

Ellington, Cleta, *Christ: The Living Water The Catholic Church in Mississippi Today.* Catholic Diocese of Jackson, Mississippi 1989.

Faust, Patricia, Editor, *Encyclopedia of the Civil War Illustrated*, New York: Harper Row 1986.

Gerow, R. O. Bishop, *Cradle Days of St. Mary's at Natchez*, Marerro: Hope Haven Press, 1941.

Healy, Sister Kathleen R.S.M. *Frances Warde, American Founder of the Sisters of Mercy*. New York: Seabury Press, 1973.

Higginson, Thomas W. *Margaret Fuller Ossoli*, New York: Chelsea House 1980.

In and About Vicksburg, A Guide to the City and Vicinity. An Anonymous Account. Gibraltar Publishing Co., 1890.

Jolly, Ellen Ryan C.C.D. *Nuns of the Battlefield*. Providence: Providence Rhode Island Visitor Press, 1927.

Leslie, Frank. *Famous Leaders & Battle Scenes of the Civil War, ed*. Louis Shepherd Moat. New York: Mrs. Frank Leslie Publisher, 1898.

Maguire, Mother M. Bernard. *The Story of the Sisters of Mercy in Mississippi*. New York: P.J. Kennedy, 1931.

Maher, Sister Mary Denis. *To Bind up the Wounds: Catholic Sister Nurses in the U.S. Civil War,* New York, Westport, Conn. London: Greenwood Press, 1989

Marszalek, John F. *Sherman A Soldier's Passion for Order*. First Vintage Civil War Library Edition, January 1994.

McLemore, Richard Aubrey. *A History of Mississippi*, Vol. I. University of Mississippi Press, Jackson, Mississippi 1973.

Memoirs of the Pittsburgh Sisters of Mercy compiled from Various Sources. 1843-1917. New York: The Devin-Adair Co., 1918.

Muldrey, Sister M. Hermenia R.S.M. *Abounding in Mercy — Mother Austin Carroll*. New Orleans: Habersham, 1988.

Pillar, James J. O.M.I. *The Catholic Church in Mississippi 1837-1965*. New Orleans: Hauser Press, 1965.

Smith, Mary Constance R.S.M., *A Sheaf of Golden Years 1856-1906, History of St. Louis Sisters of Mercy*. New York: Benziger, 1906.

Stepsis, Ursula CSA and Liptak, Dolores RSM editors of *Pioneer Healers: The History of Women Religious in American Health Care*. New York: Crossroad, 1989. Judith Metz author of chapter on Civil War Nurses.

ARCHIVES

Boeckman, Frances and Haien, Jo Ann , Archivists "Archives of Diocese of Natchez-Jackson, Mississippi" Jackson.

Curran, Emmett, S. J. "Georgetown University Archives" and *Woodstock Letters*, a Jesuit publication of Woodstock College, obituaries and information on Sumner brothers.

Freeland, Deborah, artist of sketch of University of Mississippi campus Oxford, Mississippi 1848-1906.

Harper, Sister M. Emmanuel, Archivist. "Archives of the Sisters of Mercy of Vicksburg, MS." Annals, chronicles, notes, original letters and documents, recollections of senior sisters, scrapbooks containing programs, newspaper and periodical clippings, minutes of corporation meetings, financial records, funeral home records, newspaper obituaries, Sister Ignatius Sumner's personal scrapbook, the original manuscript of the journal and the expanded journal done from dictation before Sister Ignatius died. 4 other handwritten manuscripts.

Hodge, Sister M. Patricia, Archivist. "Archives of the Sisters of Mercy in Pittsburgh, PA."

Kirsh, Sister M. Consuella, Archivist. "Archives of Sisters of Mercy Cresson, PA."

LaGarde, Glenda, booklets, exhibits of memorabilia, materials, displays, oral histories, symposium of scholars, programs for the project funded by the Mississippi Humanities Council titled St. Francis School *Cradle of the Humanities for Vicksburg 1860-1991* — a year study and involvement of the total community with LaGarde as project director of the influence of the school on the community. Much information from the Sisters of Mercy Archives Vicksburg.

Loeb, Sister M. Claude, Archivist. "Archives of Sisters of Mercy Rochester, N.Y."

McMahon, Mollie, Archivist, "Archives of Sisters of Mercy of the Americas Silver Spring, MD."

Muldrey, Sister M. Hermenia, Archivist. "Archives of Sisters of Mercy New Orleans, LA."

Mullin, Sister M. Kenneth, Archivist. "Archives of Sisters of Mercy Buffalo, N.Y."

Nolan, Charles, Archivist. "Archives of the Archdiocese of New Orleans." Letters exchanged from Sister DeSales to Archbishop Leray and information on the Howard Association and yellow fever epidemics.

Obituary Scrapbook by Charles Riles, retired funeral home director. Obituaries of each deceased, Mississippi Sister of Mercy.

O'Neill, Francis P., Reference Librarian, Maryland Historical Society Museum and Library of Maryland History, Baltimore, Maryland, information on Sumner, Steele, and Payson families and Sumner brothers.

Powers, Sister M. Felicitas, former Archivist. "Archives of Sisters of Mercy Baltimore, Maryland." Present Archivists: Sister Helen Sigrist and Irene Calahan.

Pyne, Tricia, Special Collections Lauinger Library, Georgetown University, Washington, D.C., information and obituaries of Sumner brothers.

Record Group 153 Office of Judge Advocate General (Army) Court Martial Case Files 1809-1938. File No. MM2079. Thomas Four Company D, 52nd States Colored Infantry, May 20, 1865. Major General N. J. T. Dana.

Terry, Blanche, Historian. Old Court House Museum Vicksburg, Mississippi, list of 312 names of soldiers who died in Vicksburg during the Civil War, some of whom died in the Cobb House School and Convent (St. Catherine's) and are buried in Soldiers' Rest Cemetery in Vicksburg. These records were from Frank J. Fisher Funeral Home 1860-1865.

Varga, Nicholas, Archivist. "Archives of Loyola College in Baltimore, Maryland."

ARTICLES

Bishop, Ralph, editor of pamphlets for National Endowment for the Humanities. Pamphlet: "Vicksburg's Irish." 1985.

McCloskey, Sister M. Matthew, R.S.M., *Mississippi Register: Sisters of Mercy Centennial Edition 1860-1960*, Diocese of Natchez-Jackson, Oct. 14, 1960.

Marzalek, John F. "Call to Arms," *Notre Dame Magazine*, Autumn 1992, Vol. 21, Number 3.

"Mercy Bulletin", Vol. 2:1 (Winter, 1928) p. 1. Grand Rapids, Michigan, illustrated Sister of Mercy ministering to soldier commissioned by Abraham Lincoln to White House Artist Florence Meyer.

Reddoch, Sister M. Callista, R.S.M. and Harper, Sister M. Emmanuel, R.S.M., "Vicksburg River City of Many Cultures" Pamphlet: "The Sisters of Mercy Teachers and Healers," Ralph Bishop, editor National Endowment for the Humanities project. 1985.

Roberts, Barbara, "Sisters of Mercy from Vicksburg to Shelby Springs" in *Alabama Heritage Magazine*, Editor Suzanne Wolfe, No. 11, Winter, 1989. Quarterly of the University of Alabama, Tuscaloosa, Alabama.

Spengler and Miazza family reunion booklets, sketches, oral interviews, and scrapbooks.

"A Valiant Woman," obituary and article about Mrs. Frances Allonby Sumner, probably 1882, Article intact, but dates missing from scrapbook, in *Ave Maria Magazine*.

NEWSPAPERS

Vicksburg Weekly Whig, October 27, 1860.

Vicksburg Evening Citizen, April 9, 1861; September 5, 1862; January 6, 1865; June 4, 1866.

Vicksburg Daily Herald, April 11, 12, 13, 14, 1898.

Vicksburg Evening Post, Sisters' obituaries, June 17, 1895; September 7, 1918; October & December 1876; March 9, 1910.

Vicksburg Evening Post, September 7, 1937.

Vicksburg Evening Post, December 10, 1989, letter to Post from John Loviza.

Jackson Daily Paper, May 15, 1875.

Many more articles from the Vicksburg daily papers from scrapbooks with the dates missing.

ORAL INTERVIEWS

Kathleen Brabston Cook. Descendant of Cook family in diary. A lady extremely knowledgeable of local and family history. She quoted from the journal of Minerva Hines Cook.

Gordon Cotton. Archivist Vicksburg Old Court House Museum, author, Civil War historian, local historian, expert on local history.

Karen Gamble. Journalist at *Vicksburg Evening Post* checked many names and dates from the paper.

Joe Gerache. Local pharmacist, expert on medical aspects of Civil War history. Local historian.

Christopher Kaufman, Historian and author of *Ministry and Meaning A Religious History of Catholic Health Care in the United States*. Former colleague of Sister Ethelbert Demuth.

Peter Miazza, Mary Helen Irby, Tom Spengler. Relatives attending the Miazza-Spengler family reunions. All extremely knowledgeable about local history, family and St. Peter Church history.

Ken Penhale. Shelby Springs, Alabama historian and restorer of the Shelby Springs cemetery.

Sister M. Hermenia Muldrey. Mercy expert on Mercy history, New Orleans, Louisiana.

Charles Riles. Former owner of Fisher-Riles Funeral Home, local historian, expert on local cemeteries, author, expert on obituaries of Sisters of Mercy, faithful friend to all the Sisters.

Terry Winchell. Vicksburg National Military Park guide, author, local historian, Civil War historian.

PICTURES AND ILLUSTRATION

Mary Farrell Thomas, Tupelo, Mississippi, photographer of portrait by Florence Meyer.

Sister Elise Todd, illustrator maps of Sisters' travels.

Sister Mary Paulinus Oakes, R.S.M. originally from Vicksburg, Mississippi, confesses that she is a history buff with a long interest in the Civil War and Southern history. She has a B.A. from Webster University, St. Louis and a Masters from Xavier University in Chicago and Loyola in New Orleans. She has served as elementary school principal and high school administrator and taught in Mercy schools in Mississippi and Oklahoma. For twenty years she has been on the adjunct faculty of Hinds Community College in Hinds and Warren counties teaching American Literature. During the last decade, she has been instrumental in setting up homeless shelters for wom-

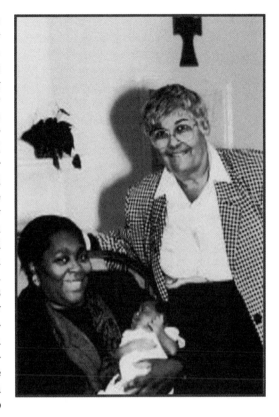

en and children in New Orleans and Jackson, Mississippi. She presently serves as certified chaplain in the chemical dependency and behaviorial health units of St. Dominic Hospital in Jackson, Mississippi.

Sister Paulinus is known for her networking. She is working on a long-range project for women and children at risk. This project will include training for life skills and GED training. It will be housed in a large thrift store Jackson area.

All proceeds from this book will benefit Mississippi Mercy Ministries with the Poor.

While leading a busy life, Sister has taken part in some of the history-making events in Mississippi. She has continually researched the Sisters of Mercy history. This book is the result of ten years research.

Index

Bruser, Mrs. W. H.   87
burning of church   21
Bury, Bessie   15, 16
Butler, Andrew, Senator South Carolina, opponent of Charles Sumner   6
Butler, General Benjamin   24, 34, 75
Byrne, Sister Camillus, Catherine McAuley's godchild and mentor of Novitiate   6, 7, 50, 59

C

Cahaba   75
Canby, Major General, Edward   32
Canton   9, 19, 43, 63, 77
Capitol building   23
Carrier, Reverend J.C.   30
Carroll, Sister Austin, Mercy historian   2, 53, 57, 62
Carroll, Charles   13
caves   16
cemetery, convent   54,66
Chamberlain, Captain   28
Charles Street, street in Baltimore   2
Chicago   10, 36
Chimneyville   21
Choctaw   11, 14, 56
Christmas Eve in Jackson 1863   19
Chunky, Mississippi   62, 63
Clinton, Mississippi   17, 95
Clinton, Mrs. Tillier   87
clothing, shortage for Sisters   21
collection of money for Sisters   32
Condon, Julia   16
Confederacy, Confererate government provided rations only,   9
Confederate Chaplains   79, 81
Confirmation   34, 37, 39, 45
consumption   36, 63
convent   37, 40, 76
convert   3, 21, 26, 33, 45, 46, 73
Cook, Jared Reese family   17, 30, 44
Cooper's Well   17, 38
Corbitt, Jane, Sister Catherine   36
Corinth, Battle of   18
Creole   24, 34, 39, 75, 80
Crimean War   xii
Crofton, Mrs. Elizabeth   87

M

N

O